Beverly Hills
Beauty Secrets

Beverly Hills
Beauty Secrets

A Prominent Dermatologist and Plastic Surgeon's Insider Guide to Facial Rejuvenation

DOUGLAS HAMILTON, MD, and
BABAK AZIZZADEH, MD

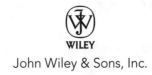

John Wiley & Sons, Inc.

Published by John Wiley & Sons, Inc., Hoboken, New Jersey
Published simultaneously in Canada

All photographs © 2009 by Douglas Hamilton, MD, and Babak Azizzadeh, MD. The illustration on page 13 is from *Master Techniques in Facial Rejuvenation* by Babak Azizzadeh, Mark Murphy, and Calvin M. Johnson Jr.

The information contained in this book is not intended to serve as a replacement for professional medical advice. Any use of the information in this book is at the reader's discretion. The author and the publisher specifically disclaim any and all liability arising directly or indirectly from the use or application of any information contained in this book. A health care professional should be consulted regarding your specific situation.

For general information about our other products and services, please contact our Customer Care Department within the United States at (800) 762-2974, outside the United States at (317) 572-3993 or fax (317) 572-4002.

Wiley also publishes its books in a variety of electronic formats. Some content that appears in print may not be available in electronic books. For more information about Wiley products, visit our web site at www.wiley.com.

Library of Congress Cataloging-in-Publication Data:

Hamilton, Douglas, date.
  Beverly Hills beauty secrets : a prominent dermatologist and plastic surgeon's insider guide to facial rejuvenation / Douglas Hamilton and Babak Azizzadeh.
      p. cm.
  Includes index.
  ISBN 978-0-470-29403-1 (cloth: alk. paper)
1. Surgery, Plastic. 2. Face—Surgery. 3. Face—Care and hygiene.
I. Azizzadeh, Babak. II. Title.
  RD119.5.F33H346 2009
  617.9'5--dc22
                                                                    2008055948

Printed in the United States of America

10   9   8   7   6   5   4   3   2   1

To my loving wife and life partner, Jessica. Her inner and outer beauty inspires me. Thank you for coming into my life! To my extraordinary children, Kylie and Logan—their smiles and hugs rejuvenate me. To my parents, Yafa and Habib, for their enduring love and support. To my sister, Katrin, for continually encouraging her little brother. Last but not least, to my amazing patients for allowing me to make a small difference in their lives.

—Babak Azizzadeh

To my wonderful children, Branden and Britney, who have filled my life with joy: in my heart you will remain forever young. To the memory of my parents, Charlotte and William, which will never grow old. Finally, to the patients who have given me the privilege of receiving their trust.

—Douglas Hamilton

Contents

Introduction

Forget Wall Street—Our Insider Trading Secrets Come Straight from Rodeo Drive!

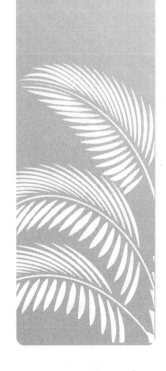

The boomers are aging—and don't want to look it.

Women are looking to nonsurgical procedures—and loving it.

Men are using beauty products—and not afraid to admit it.

We are a nation obsessed with appearance—and the statistics prove it.

According to the American Society for Aesthetic Plastic Surgery (ASAPS), Americans spent approximately $12.4 billion on cosmetic procedures in 2007. This means that more doctors than ever before are performing more procedures on more people, creating an inherent confusion about not only which procedures are the most appropriate but also which doctor is the most qualified to perform them.

It doesn't help to clarify matters that in the past decade, techniques to enhance the appearance of the face have grown exponentially. New technology makes surgery simpler and recovery faster. New products mean new brand names, and new brand names mean new buzzwords, which cause even more confusion. (Can you say "Radiesse, Restylane, and Thermage, with a side of Artefill for good measure"?)

Many of the latest techniques in cosmetic advancement involve nonsurgical procedures. In fact, recent statistics reveal a widening gap in the surgical versus nonsurgical conundrum: of the nearly 11.5 million surgical and nonsurgical procedures performed in the United States in 2007, surgical procedures accounted for only 19 percent of the total procedures, and nonsurgical procedures made up the other 81 percent.

The top five nonsurgical cosmetic procedures in 2005 were as follows:

1. Botox injections
2. Laser hair removal
3. Hyaluronic acids (Hylaform, Restylane)
4. Microdermabrasion
5. Chemical peels

Simultaneously, the demand for facial rejuvenation and beauty preservation has increased at an unprecedented rate because of increasing societal acceptance of cosmetic procedures. Popular magazines continue to tout the "youth is power" message through glossy photographs of young, unblemished, wrinkle-free models. Television has also had a huge impact: *Extreme Makeover* and *Dr. 90210* and their countless spin-offs made cosmetic surgery fodder for "reality TV" shows, and *Queer Eye for the Straight Guy* turned beauty products for men into a fad that became a trend that continues as a habit today.

As a result, a significant amount of confusion has surfaced about the cornucopia of procedures, physician board certification, cost, and the validity of "lunchtime makeovers." The trends are actually as surprising to physicians as they have been to patients. For decades surgery was performed in a medical center and nonsurgical procedures were performed at clinics, but recent statistics reveal newly emerging trends: of all the cosmetic procedures performed in 2005, 48.3 percent were performed in office-based facilities, 27.9 percent were performed in freestanding ambulatory surgical centers, and 23.8 percent were performed in hospitals.

The Best Source for Your Information

Traditionally, plastic surgeons and dermatologists were the experts who clarified the appropriate intervention to address an individual's concerns. Today, however, the Internet as well as the print media and television have become important sources of information for people who are seeking the appropriate procedure and available intervention.

Advertisements by physicians and the makers of cosmetic products and procedures are abundant. Numerous books have also been published about beauty and health, but most of the advice in these books is limited by the experience and specialty of the physicians. Despite the significant amount of available information, people seem to be more confused than ever, and most do not think that they have an unbiased source for information on facial enhancement and preservation.

That's about to change with the publication of this book. To our knowledge, this is the first book written by both a facial plastic surgeon and a dermatologist with expertise in facial rejuvenation. This groundbreaking dual expertise allows for a broad-based—and unbiased—approach to facial rejuvenation.

A mixture of excitement and concern has energized us to write this book. With the proper application of the technological and surgical approaches that are now available, many elements of facial aging can be addressed today in ways that were not imaginable even just five years ago. Nevertheless, with this advancing tide of technology and surgery comes some muddying of the waters.

The promises provided by these advances can be nullified by

their inappropriate application in unqualified hands. This can range from doctors who are far removed from their specialties, with backgrounds as slight as a weekend course certificate, to nonphysicians who are employed in a business model in which medical professionalism has been suffocated by the drive to profit.

For individuals who seek to enhance and preserve their facial appearance, our goal in writing this book is to give "insider trading" tips of which most cosmetic health care providers are aware. These include the following:

- Providing the guidelines for understanding the aging changes that are specific to the face so that individuals can be educated about alternative treatments
- Clarifying the available surgical and nonsurgical treatments
- Providing the all-important criteria for choosing the physician specialist who would understand the appropriate procedure

Together, we have more than four decades of experience in facial plastic surgery and dermatology, all of which is poured into this book. Through a combination of sound advice, quantifiable research, unvarnished truth, and actual case studies from our two practices, we want to enable the reader to choose a life-enhancing result with money well spent—and hope and trust well placed. That is our sincere wish.

1

Beauty
More Than Just Skin Deep?

The best and most beautiful things in the world cannot be seen, nor touched . . . but are felt in the heart.

—HELEN KELLER

What is beauty? Is it entirely "in the eye of the beholder," as the saying goes? Is it something we can measure, test, rate, and evaluate objectively? Can you solve it with math, science, or physics? Is it subjective, quantifiable, or even worth pursuing?

Throughout history—and even today—each country, continent, or civilization has defined beauty in its own unique way. Open any copy of *National Geographic* and you will see beauty in all its various forms; facial and body modification, tattoos, piercings, and other depictions of unconventional (to us, anyway) beauty leap off the page.

How do we feel when we see bones piercing ears and necks elongated from a dozen brass rings that have been worn since birth? That is why it is said that "beauty is in the eye of the beholder." What is beautiful to some is shocking to others—and vice versa.

As children, we know little of beauty. Our parents are beautiful, our siblings are beautiful, our own reflections are beautiful. It is only when we enter the so-called real world that the social structure can affect our own perceptions of beauty.

According to a study published in the June 2001 issue of *Archives of Dermatology*, many factors go into our self-perception of beauty:

> Ironically, most people seem unable to accurately judge their own attractiveness. Correlations between self-ratings and objective measures of individual attractiveness are remarkably low. . . . Only high self-ratings of physical attractiveness are generated among those with relatively greater self-esteem, emotional stability, and capacity for dominance. Favorable ratings by others are more likely when the individual being rated has good social skills and is not self-conscious. Popular, sexually experienced people are rated as attractive by both themselves and others.

Clearly, those who feel more beautiful tend to rate themselves as more attractive. Where does this positive self-perception come from—and how can the rest of us get it? Quite often, the societies we live in dictate what most of us perceive as perfection or beauty. The handsome athlete, the supermodel, the square-jawed actor, and the blond actress are the images with which we in modern America are bombarded every day. After such constant bombardment, it is almost inevitable that we eventually come to see them as beautiful. Yet only rarely do we stop to realize that these celebrities are in the minority, not the majority, that they are the exception, not the norm.

Although we may sugarcoat such findings with laboratories and press releases, the research indicates that we are not as far removed from our Neanderthal ancestors as we like to think.

Attractive features meant that a couple was more likely to reproduce; more reproduction meant more children; more children meant that a society was more likely to survive.

Can beauty be that simple and that prehistoric? Even now, dressed in bangles and bows and buffed with Bowflex, can we still be responding to the primal urges that tell us that a more beautiful person is likely to be a more healthy person or a better mating, hunting, or life partner? Does our quest for beauty really come down to nothing more than wanting to be with someone who is more likely to succeed in surviving, hunting, and gathering than all the other Average Joes and Janes at the bus stop?

Scientific studies indicate that from its very beginning, the ideal of beauty has always been about fertility and the survival of the species. The specimens who were deemed most beautiful often found the most mates, leading to more offspring and the notion of "survival of the fittest." This is no less true in humans than it is in animals, for whom various stripes or plumage signify a more attractive, and thus more highly desirable, mate.

What "plumage" did the ancients prefer? How do different cultures view beauty? Research indicates that in every culture—regardless of race, religion, or geographic region—there is a preference by men for women with full lips, clean skin, lustrous hair, good muscle tone, a youthful gait, animated facial expressions, and a high energy level.

As for the qualities that women want in their mates, facial symmetry seems as important as body size. Although ancient women viewed large pectoral muscles and biceps as desirable weapons of war, it has also been discovered that in modern times, men with symmetrical faces have sex four years earlier than their asymmetrical counterparts and have two to three times as many partners during their sexual prime.

"What Is Beautiful Is Good"

The Greek poet Sappho once wrote, "What is beautiful is good, and who is good will soon be beautiful." Since then, much has been written about beauty and, not surprisingly, Sappho's quote has proven to be quite astute—at least the first part, "What is beautiful is good." Indeed, from better grades to more room on the sidewalk, the people we consider to be more attractive receive preferential treatment in almost every area of life.

In an article in the July 1983 issue of the *American Journal of Sociology,* authors Murray Webster and James E. Driskell combine several previous studies to determine that "the most general conclusion from research is that the world must be a more pleasant and satisfying place for attractive people because they possess almost all types of social advantages that can be measured."

Which social advantages are they referring to, exactly? The authors catalog myriad such advantages, beginning as early as childhood: "Attractive schoolchildren are expected by their teachers to achieve higher school marks than unattractive children, and they usually do so; their misdemeanors are judged less serious and it is predicted that they will have more successful careers."

Attractive children often grow up to become attractive adults, and the benefits continue to multiply: "Attractive adults are thought to have happier marriages than those who are unattractive, and that expectation seems to be fulfilled. Opinions of attractive adults are more likely to be agreed with; attractive adults are perceived as having better mental health. Attractive adults are even granted larger 'personal space' on the sidewalk than are the unattractive."

Supermodel Tyra Banks once wore a hidden camera while wearing a fat suit, and it was amazing at how differently she was treated compared to when the suit came off, but research reveals that what she experienced was not an isolated event. Studies prove that thin, attractive people really do earn more money and become more successful—in business and in love—than those who are heavier and considered unattractive.

For example, a 2005 study by the Federal Reserve Bank of St. Louis reports that "good-looking, slim, tall people tend to make more money than their plain-Jane counterparts."

Writing in the December 2002 issue of the *Journal of Young Investigators,* author Charles Feng from Stanford University states, "Psychological research suggests that people generally choose mates with a similar level of attractiveness. The evolutionary theory is that by mating with someone who has similar genes, one's own genes are conserved. Moreover, a person's demeanor and personality also influences how others perceive his or her beauty."

Furthermore, an article by Murad Alam and Jeffrey Dover in the June 2001 issue of *Archives of Dermatology* boasts research to support the theory that

> the best-looking women in high school are 10 times as likely to marry as the least attractive, and they are more likely to marry sooner and marry persons of greater wealth or social status. Sexual encounters are more numerous and varied for attractive people. Better treatment for the better looking extends to the workplace. West Point graduates with facial features more suggestive of dominance are more likely to achieve high rank. In the private sector, the good-looking are more likely to be hired, given a higher salary, and promoted sooner.

Youth and Beauty

Some people say that youth is beauty. Research indicates that this truism may be more accurate than we ever imagined. Anthropologist Doug Jones studied the subject of youth—or *neoteny*, which means the "retention of some larval or immature characters in adulthood"—in five populations: Brazilians, Americans, Russians, the Aché Indians of Paraguay, and the Hiwi Indians of Venezuela. The study, which was published in the journal *Current Anthropology*, found "cross-cultural evidence that males . . . show an attraction to females with neotenous facial proportions (a combination of large eyes, small noses and full lips) even after female age is controlled for."

Youth and beauty often go hand in hand. Our baby boomer patients almost always mention the words "more youthful" when describing their ideal appearance. Youth is truly fleeting, and there are qualities of youthful skin—its fleshiness, glow, tone, color, and tautness—that have an expiration date as we age.

Alam and Dover, in their June 2001 article in *Archives of Dermatology*, seem to conclude that age is indeed a grave concern for those who seek to define or recapture their own sense of beauty:

> Ratings of physical attractiveness decline with advancing age for both men and women, with the decrease more steep for women. Older women are regarded as less feminine. Those who appear aged beyond their years complain of being repeatedly told that they look tired or unwell. As Ambrose Phillips poignantly observed, "The flowers anew, returning seasons bring! But beauty faded has no second spring."

It is also true that we live in a youth-oriented society. Most movies are targeted to the young, magazines feature younger and younger models, and beauty products specifically target the youth market. In many instances, the word *aging* itself is considered less than appealing. Nevertheless, the definition of beauty remains elusive.

"I believe being beautiful is a double-edged sword," says Leslie G. Christin, the founder and creative force behind Cara Cosmetics International, "as I'm more critical of 'beauty' compared to someone in another field. Of course, I can make someone look beautiful—yet in TV and film you are not allowed to look bad, unless it is a character role." She notes, "We define an actress on how old they look."

The "beauty" of living in modern times means that through very simple procedures or readily available products, the glow and radiance of youth can be achieved—within reason. Simply by using various creams and lotions and following a daily home regimen, people can often achieve a more youthful beauty in a matter of weeks or months, without surgery or other costly procedures. What they gain in return is more confidence—and that in itself is beauty personified.

Face Value

When it comes to the human face, the definition of beauty is elusive. We often hear patients who are not that far out of their forties—or even their thirties—complaining, "I just don't feel beautiful anymore." (What they really seem to be saying is, "Make me young again!")

Many of us answer that call any way we know how, by using our professions to help our patients feel better on the inside *and* the outside. This may be one reason that Americans today spend more money on beauty products than they do on social services or education. Nevertheless, the question "What is beautiful?" confounds us.

What, then, is beauty?

Of course, there is physical beauty, which we see from the outside. Yet as cultures and cliques change, so too does our definition of beauty. The plump Rubenesque beauties of seventeenth- and eighteenth-century Europe have given way to the current chant of "thin is in." What of the face, however? Can the size of your facial features play a role in your perceived beauty to others and, possibly, yourself?

According to a study by Karl Grammer and Randy Thornhill on human facial attractiveness and sexual selection, published in the 1994 *Journal of Comparative Psychology*, the answer could be yes. Grammer and Thornhill claim, "The human face contains . . . facial features that develop or increase in size at puberty. . . . Enlarged jaws, chins, and cheekbones in men are examples of facial secondary sexual traits that are influenced by testosterone . . . largeness in these features are considered sexually attractive because of advertised immunocompetence."

So where do all these studies, quotes, and experts leave us? In our clinical practices, our focus is to improve areas on the face that stand out and detract attention from the eyes. The eyes should be the focus of the face, especially in social interactions. Features that are out of proportion to the rest of the face tend to draw the focus away from the eyes and create an imbalance to the face.

For instance, a large bulbous nose, sagging jowls, angry frown lines, and poor skin quality all tend to be distracting features. Using the latest in technology and computer simulation, we can now more clearly reveal what someone would look like after surgery; making side-by-side comparisons of before and after photos, we then decide together what the most ideal and natural outcome would be. People are often surprised by how even small changes can have a significant impact on one's youthfulness and beauty.

Beauty Is Harmony

"Beauty is harmony." So says the noted maxillofacial surgeon, Dr. Stephen Marquardt, who has even created a scientific method of defining beauty to prove his theory.

After years of studying beauty in a variety of cultures and eras, from ancient times right up to the present, Dr. Marquardt concluded that the groups in question worship basically the same perceptions of facial beauty. Here is how he arrived at this conclusion:

> We computer-analyzed photos of thousands of "attractive" faces from every geographic race on the planet. This analysis included a deconstruction of these faces to determine their precise geometric constitution and how these faces differed mathematically from average and unattractive faces. We then applied hundreds of geometric algorithms to the faces to determine a mathematic and geometric commonality between these images. Ultimately, this led to the construction of an entire series of unique geometric forms, which appeared to "predict" high attractiveness or "beauty." We called these unique geometric forms "Archetypal Facial Mask Templates" or "Masks."

This sounds convincing, but can any equation based on hard measurements and empirical science really define something as esoteric and elusive as beauty? Or is it up to each individual to determine what beauty is—within oneself and about others?

In the course of his studies, Dr. Marquardt developed and patented the "beauty mask." This mask is a result of his cultural surveys on beauty and, according to Dr. Marquardt, reflects the fact that all groups have an international standard of beauty.

What Dr. Marquardt calls the Golden Proportion drives the construct of the mask: all the defining angles and features of a beautiful face—eyes, nose, brow, forehead, cheeks, and chin—are proportionate to one another.

The doctor explains, "With the use of mathematics, computers, and massive databases of 'attractive' faces, we have been able to quantify facial attractiveness in a consistent mathematical computer model." There are different masks for men and women, but both are built on the mathematical equations and the database of attractive faces.

Amazingly, this mask aligns perfectly with beautiful faces throughout the ages, from Queen Nefertiti to Marilyn Monroe

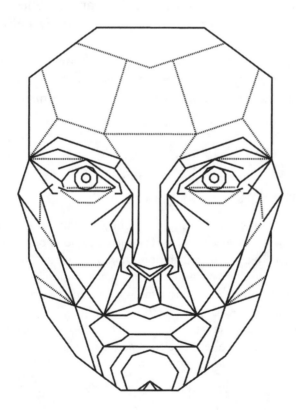

The Marquardt adult female beauty mask

to Elizabeth Hurley. The mask is a perfect mathematic and geometric creation, and no biological system, or face, is perfect. However, the more closely any face fits the mask, the more beautiful it will be judged to be by other humans. Dr. Marquardt states that he has never found a face that is perceived as highly attractive or beautiful that does not closely correlate with the form of the mask.

When It Comes to Beauty, *You* Are the Beholder

We concede that, like harmony, beauty is a pleasing notion that's equally hard to define. What of inner beauty, however? We all know that even though it's hard to define, inner beauty is often as obvious as outer beauty. There are people who not only look more beautiful because of the passions and emotions they hold inside, they also make us feel prettier just by being in their presence.

We are often introduced to people who are not attractive on the outside, according to social norms; however, after spending a few minutes with them, we realize their inner beauty. This

A QUEST FOR BEAUTY: COSMETIC SURGERY FOR MEN

The American Society for Aesthetic Plastic Surgery recently conducted a survey and discovered that 10 percent of nonsurgical and surgical cosmetic procedures are being performed on men. This represents a more than 300 percent increase since 1997 in the number of cosmetic procedures performed on men, and it shows that men are becoming much more comfortable with using plastic surgery to look their best.

Procedures popular among male clients include eye lifts (blepharoplasty), nose jobs (rhinoplasty), and nonsurgical options such as BOTOX Cosmetic, laser hair-reduction treatments, and skin-resurfacing treatments.

inner beauty can instantly overpower outer features. Conversely, we often meet so-called physically beautiful people, such as actors or models, with whom we spend enough time to realize that they are so lacking inside, it begins to diminish their outer beauty.

In our offices, we see beauty constantly. There are the classic beauties we can spot instantly, such as actors and actresses, models, or hosts and hostesses; they fit the very narrow definition of beauty as it applies to height, weight, skin, hair, and symmetry. Then there are the radiant beauties who defy convention yet still manage to be attractive through a variety of demonstrable features such as athleticism, enthusiasm, fitness, and overall health. Finally, there are the hard-to-define beauties, those whose inner beauty radiates throughout and not only overshadows their physical imperfections but makes one forget about the very qualities they are coming to correct.

We chose to write this chapter on youth and beauty for one simple reason: most people who come to us want to feel more beautiful or recapture their youth. You might be coming to this book with the same sentiments. If we were to equate one single word with beauty, it would be *confidence*. Above and beyond all the physical parameters, measurements, and definitions that we can apply to physical beauty itself, it all comes down to this: those patients who walk into—or out of—our offices feeling more self-confident than ever before are resonating the meaning of true beauty, in our opinion.

As physicians, we listen to the patient first—and counsel second. Far from fitting the stereotype of Beverly Hills dermatologists and plastic surgeons who counsel "more, more, more," we often counter with "less is more."

After all, what a patient often thinks is an imperfection can actually be a huge part of his or her charm. The best part about our job is that we serve only to make the patient happy. In our one-on-one consultations, we discuss all options: surgical and nonsurgical, extreme and casual, temporary and permanent. Each patient receives a specific diagnosis because each patient is a unique individual.

Now you know what we can do to make you more beautiful,

but what can *you* do? Can what you do influence how people think you look? Can what you do influence how *you* think you look? Research seems to indicate that the most effective method of self-beautification is also the easiest and the cheapest: smile.

According to a 1999 article in the *European Journal of Social Psychology*, "it was found that smiling increased rated attractiveness when compared to a non-smiling neutral expression. . . . It was also demonstrated that smiling subjects were attributed greater degrees of sincerity, sociability, and competence."

Self-confidence is true beauty.

A report in the February 1984 issue of the *Journal of Personality and Social Psychology* reiterates these findings: "Target persons were less attractive when posing sad expressions than when posing neutral or happy expressions, which did not differ. . . . Both facial and bodily attractiveness were predictive of overall attractiveness, but the face was a slightly more powerful predictor."

That's good news, because confidence is internal, not external. Yet you feel it when you see it, and this is where we often come into play. Everyone has physical imperfections that he or she would like to improve. Our goal with our patients is to help them feel better about themselves and, in the process, more confident.

Today, tomorrow, and the next day, you are already a wholly unique and beautiful individual. What can we do to make you more beautiful? The answer is equally simple: make you feel more confident.

2

Conquer the Consultation

Deciding What to Change

Lasers, peels, face-lifts, eyelid lifts, rhinoplasty, Botox—so many options and so much confusion. Facial analysis is the cornerstone in deciding what the appropriate treatment is for your particular concerns. Only after an appropriate analysis can we provide the ideal treatment. This chapter is designed to help you see your face in a much more analytical manner. After all, you are here to explore, discover, and, we hope, uncover the secrets to dozens of your most burning questions about the human face.

We can tell you with confidence that even if we haven't personally met you yet, we've seen you before. The human face is our medium for obtaining ideal results for people of many ages, ethnicities, and socioeconomic statuses and with all sorts of problems. One of the greatest things we can offer our patients is familiarity with their concerns. Every day, we see people who want to improve their appearance, and now we will turn our full attention to you.

Our readers, like our patients, are individuals with individual needs. Some questions to ponder include the following:

- What do you want to change about your face?
- Why are you reading this book?
- What made you pick it up? Was it something that happened in the last few years or something that's been nagging at you your entire life?
- What can we do to help?
- What knowledge can we impart?

In this chapter we will discuss the following key elements to answer the universal question, "What would you like to change about your face?" They include the following:

- The "Quick, If You Could Change Just One Thing, What Would It Be?" test
- The diagnosis
- Our facial analysis
- The Rejuvenation Equation Quiz: Ten Quick Questions to Help You Get from A to Easy!
- The consultation

These vital sections will help both of us to understand why, what, when, and how you want to go about changing your face. It's not a simple question, we know. We see people struggle with it every day, but the more information we can provide, the easier that struggle becomes.

The following sections will help you to understand what a professional consultation with a dermatologist or a facial plastic surgeon must entail.

The "Quick, If You Could Change Just One Thing, What Would It Be?" Test

The most important person in the process of facial rejuvenation is you. You are the only one who matters, and your concerns are of utmost importance.

If you're being honest, you'll know right away what you'd change about your face. (If you're *really* being honest, you knew the minute you saw the title of this section.) There are areas that are overlooked by most individuals when they analyze their own faces, such as brow drooping and small chins. However, no one knows your face the way you do. Even your mother or your spouse, as often as they look at your face, won't know it the way you do.

The road to facial rejuvenation always starts with the diagnosis. Once the diagnosis is established, the therapy is naturally born.

Thus, ask yourself the question, then answer it. That's all you have to do—for now. Later in this chapter, we'll have a more conclusive quiz to help fine-tune your answers as well as your reasons for having aesthetic enhancements in the first place.

LET'S TALK ABOUT LIP AUGMENTATION

Improvement and enlargement of lip contour is commonly desired. There are multiple ways to approach this goal. The treatment options include the following:

1. Hyaluronic acids: Juvéderm, Restylane
2. Collagen: Cosmoplast, Cosmoderm, Evolence Breeze (pending FDA approval)
3. Lip implants: Gore-Tex (SoftForm), AlloDerm, VeraFil (not FDA approved for this area; used off-label)
4. Fat grafting
5. Silicone (not FDA approved for this area; used off-label)
6. Cymetra

Hyaluronic acids and collagen products are currently the most commonly used methods for lip augmentation.

The Diagnosis: What's Going On?

This chapter is about your face: what you like about it, what you don't, what you'd change if you could, and what you wouldn't. It's natural to have strong feelings about one's own face. Hair may dull and gray, arms and legs get bigger and smaller, breasts and buttocks change shape, but our faces are forever—or so it would seem. That's because the thing we see every day is hard to see objectively. It's kind of like watching a trickle of water turn a valley into a gorge and then into a canyon over years and years of erosion. Unfortunately, that's just what happens to our faces over time; they erode.

As much as we'd like to avoid it—and as hard as we work to prevent it—age happens, whether we like it or not. Age also changes us. From top to bottom, your entire face is affected by age. For instance, your forehead may furrow and host a series of creases. Your brows can droop. The skin around the eyes is sensitive and thin; changes here range from wrinkling to sagging to bags to a puffiness that never seems to go away. Even your nose can seem longer and more "hooked" as it droops with the gaining years.

Loose facial skin can create jowls; lips can grow thinner and more discolored with each passing year. The chin grows weaker, at least in appearance, due to the erosion of the jaw bone and the loss of chin fat. Then there are the ravages of sun damage over time.

It all happens slowly, minutely, taking days and weeks and months and years, until the changes are so noticeable they can no longer be ignored. That is why so many people tell us, "I don't know what happened; one morning I just woke up and looked old!"

That's when they take the path to our office. One day you too might take the path to your doctor's office. What will you find when you get there? What are the first steps, and how can anyone help you to find the face you're looking for if you're not sure where to start?

The road to facial rejuvenation always starts with the diagnosis. Once the diagnosis is established, the therapy is naturally born. It's a two-part process, like washing your face before you dry it or drying it before you put on your makeup. You simply can't do one without the other, yet so many people try by making assumptions about how quick and easy some procedures are or how severe or simple their problems may be.

In many ways this book is a how-to, self-help guide to learning all there is to know about your face. We are simply trying to give you as much material and provide as much knowledge as we can before you take the next logical step, which is consulting a medical professional.

In evaluating the aging face one may see aesthetic changes in four broad terms: laxity (type A), furrowing (type B), rhytids (type C), and facial atrophy—facial volume loss—(type D). (See the illustrations at right.) Rhytids are superficial wrinkles, whereas furrows are deeper, valleylike expression lines.

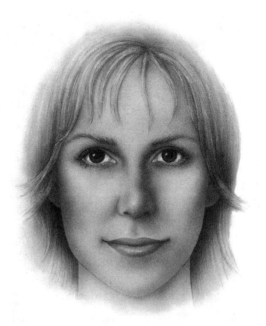

Age: 30s

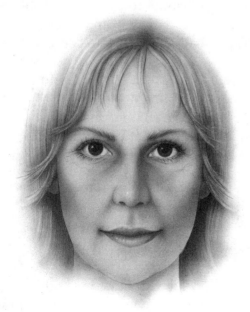

Age: 40s

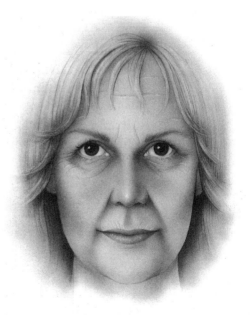

Age: Early 60s

Other factors that contribute to an aging appearance are color irregularity and loss of skin luster. The interplay among various aging processes often makes it impossible to obtain a complete therapeutic effect from any one modality.

Two examples are the marionette folds that remain below the corner of the mouth after face-lift procedures and the poor resolution of crow's feet around the eyes after laser resurfacing. Every face is unique in its elements of aging, and every area may have several pathologies that contribute to the aging problem. The marionette folds and crow's feet have complex etiologies and therefore require several modalities in order to address them appropriately.

As a result, noninvasive techniques are of great value for some aging defects but not for others. Skin and muscle laxity of more than a moderate degree requires surgical intervention, whereas fine rhytids, furrowing, and volume loss are preferably treated by lasers and noninvasive injectables, either separately or in combination.

Our Facial Analysis: Diagnosis Leads Simply to Treatment

We will fully discuss the many available treatments on the market today in subsequent chapters, and we will have much more to say about your initial consultation in this chapter. No matter what the treatment or when the consultation occurs, however, make sure that you are clear about everything your doctor is telling you. If something stumps you, ask a question. If something still stumps you, ask more questions.

HOW TO KNOW YOUR DOCTOR KNOWS (IS HE OR SHE UP TO DATE?)

It's hard for many cosmetic specialists to keep current with technology and techniques. Here is a step-by-step procedure to help you make sure that your doctor is up-to-date.

- Confirm board certification in any one of the following:
  1. American Board of Dermatology (www.abderm.org)
  2. American Board of Facial Plastic and Reconstructive Surgery (www.abfprs.org)
  3. American Board of Plastic Surgery (www.abplsurg.org)
  4. American Board of Otolaryngology (www.aboto.org)
  5. American Board of Ophthalmology (www.abop.org)
- Confirm society and academy memberships:
  1. American Society for Dermatologic Surgery (www.asds-net.org)
  2. American Academy of Facial Plastic and Reconstructive Surgery (www.aafprs.org)
  3. American Society of Plastic Surgeons (www.plasticsurgery.org)
  4. American Society for Aesthetic Plastic Surgery (www.surgery.org)
  5. American Society of Ophthalmic Plastic and Reconstructive Surgery (www.asoprs.org)
- Determine board-certified specialty associations for the above fields (for dermasurgery, for example, it would be the American Society for Dermatologic Surgery).
- Determine committee membership in the different academies and societies: these specialty committees (such as New Technologies or Liposuction) are the recognized experts in these procedures.
- The surgical specialist should have operating privileges for the procedures that you are seeking at an accredited hospital.
- Find out about their education and surgical training.

The doctor-patient relationship is a democracy, not a dictatorship; treat it as such. Remember, this is your face—forever. Although many of the advances in dermatology and plastic surgery have made the majority of these procedures safe and effective, nothing is foolproof, and not every one is right for you.

That's what the diagnosis, analysis, and consultation are for: deciding which procedure is right for you—and why. If you understand only one part of that equation—be it the "which" or the "why"—you're not ready to have the procedure. It's just that simple.

It's easy to become intimidated by the man or woman in the white coat. Doctors' offices are sacred places, quiet and serious, but don't let the wall charts and the "medicalese" intimidate you. You are paying for the privilege of our time, expertise, attention, and, most of all, advice. So get your money's worth!

You wouldn't pay for half a box of cereal or one hour of a movie, would you? So why would you settle for anything other than full disclosure with your plastic surgeon or dermatologist?

The Rejuvenation Equation Quiz: Ten Quick Questions to Help You Get from A to Easy!

Although we work in the most cosmetic surgery–aware city in the most rejuvenation-friendly state on the planet, we realize that not everybody eats, sleeps, and breathes cosmetic surgery and aesthetic medicine. We have therefore compiled what we call a Rejuvenation Equation Quiz, a quick ten-question survey to help you ask—and answer—the uppermost questions on your mind as well as ours.

After all, this is a big decision, no matter how major or minor the product or procedure. Whether the choice is lasers or Botox or a mini-face-lift, people's conceptions of these procedures are often misconceptions, so we want you to understand not only the facts and terminology but also your reasons for making the decision to have the work done.

So sit back, relax, and answer the questions. Don't worry; nobody but you will ever read this, and there are no preconceived answers to circle or any scores to keep. This is merely a comprehensive quiz to guide you into answering some pretty serious and vital questions on your feelings about plastic surgery and dermatology—and your need for either or both in the coming years. Once you've answered each question, we'll analyze why you might have answered the way you did and what most people have to say about the matter.

Question 1: How Young Do I Want to Look?

Is your answer five years? Ten? Twenty? Thirty? There is no wrong answer, of course, only the realization that technology has its limits—and so do we. We would love to be in our twenties and even our thirties again—many people would give everything to be in their forties or fifties again—but this isn't always possible.

Anyone who promises you that you can look twenty to thirty years younger is probably anticipating a procedure so severe that not only will it *not* produce such audacious results, it will probably make you look weird rather than younger.

We will talk later about the various hallmarks of aging—tightness and a "surprised" look are not two of them. For now, however, just know that we always recommend a gradual, and gradually noticeable, regimen of a combination of surgical and nonsurgical procedures so that you always look natural, no matter what your age.

Thus, instead of asking "How young can you make me look?" at your initial consultation with a treating physician, a much better question might be "Can you make me look *refreshed*?"

Question 2: Is There a Specific Feature— Nose, Cheeks, Brow—That Is Causing Me to Consider Facial Rejuvenation?

Has something been bothering you since childhood, like chubby cheeks or a long nose? Many times it is one of these "unsightly" features—or so says an unthinking family member, friend, lover, or colleague—that propels us to seek facial rejuvenation. Sometimes you have been upset about the feature since childhood; other times it didn't bother you until a certain age, when the feature became more prominent.

Wanting a procedure is never right or wrong. We want you to look your best, at any age. Generally speaking, features that stand out, such as a big or hooked nose, large bags under the eyes, or drooping neck skin, are the ones that people inquire about all the time.

Question 3: What Procedures Do I Think Would Be Necessary to Achieve These Results?

We have people in our office all the time who come armed with great knowledge about aesthetic medicine. They are well informed; they may have read an article in *Vogue* or scoured multiple Web sites to learn about the newest and greatest procedures promising "instant results" and to "take years off your age."

When you come in for a consultation to see if those procedures are appropriate for you, it is our job to educate you about your research and to inform you about your choices. That is what the initial consultation is for.

So don't throw out what you know. Simply proceed with an open mind and take it from us that every face is unique, so there is no one pat answer or solution for every problem. With your face, your knowledge, good questions, and straight answers, we will work together to make you look years younger and feel much better.

Question 4: What Can I (Realistically) Expect to Achieve If I Have Lots of Skin Damage Due to Smoking, Drinking, Poor Nutrition, or Exposure to the Sun?

We wish more people would ask this question. Although some skin damage is difficult to treat, you can usually achieve amazing results—and a great deal of success—by talking openly and honestly with your treating physician about both your concerns and the realistic chances for significant results.

The outcome will depend on how much work you put into the process. It will be like taking care of your teeth; you cannot just see your dentist every six months for a cleaning and hope that you will have no cavities. You have to brush and floss every day as well.

Similarly, you will need to take care of your skin on a daily basis with lotions and potions recommended by your physician; you will also need routine visits with your physician and aesthetician for "skin cleaning" with lasers and peels. We will give you the details in the upcoming chapters.

Question 5: What about Genetics? Will Looking at My Parents Help Me to See My Future?

The answer to this question is yes! Both nature and nurture have a tremendous impact on the aging process. *Nurture* refers to our habits and experiences, such as smoking, sun exposure, illnesses, diet, and exercise. *Nature* refers to our genes.

Genetics plays a crucial role in determining not only what we look like but also how we age. We often find it useful when people bring in pictures of themselves throughout the years as well as pictures of their parents and siblings throughout the years. Looking at your father's heavy brow or your mother's wrinkles can help us to understand and prepare for how you will age.

Question 6: Do I Know the Difference between Fantasy and Reality?

This is not a trick question. Many people come to us wanting a particular celebrity's head on their body. Seriously—it happens all the time. However, science is not (yet) so advanced that this is possible.

Fortunately, we think that improving what you already have is a much more realistic and sensible goal than changing everything about you to resemble someone you might not even want to look like in five or ten years.

Question 7: Am I Doing This for Me— or Someone Else?

Your motives for cosmetic surgery and/or facial rejuvenation must be pure, not cloudy or ulterior. You must want to undergo these procedures for yourself—that is, to feel better about yourself. When people have procedures to please a parent, a mate, a friend, or an employer, the result can sometimes be disappointing—for both parties.

These are important issues to be discussed during your consultation with your physician. You must search within yourself to discover why, exactly, you are having this procedure done and, more important, for whom. Our philosophy is that you should always do it for yourself, never for someone else.

Question 8: Is This the Right Time for Me to Have This, or Any, Procedure?

When it comes to facial rejuvenation, timing is everything. Looking naturally beautiful and youthful requires the right combination of products and procedures at the right time so that the job gets done before it's too late and nothing looks too severe.

Despite everything, the timing will depend on you. You must be ready psychologically and physically to have these procedures. Some individuals are not ready to get started on skin care; others want to undergo major surgery without major trepidation. Most important, discuss your concerns with your physician so that together you can decide the right time that fits your needs.

Question 9: Do I Have a Strong Support System at Home?

Support is vital for the potential cosmetic surgery or dermatology patient. Regardless of how independent you may be—or just think you are—there will be recovery time, and there will be a need for someone to drive you to the office, wait around, and take you home.

There may also be a need for someone to stay with you for twenty-four to seventy-two hours, monitoring your progress, changing your bandages, or simply helping you to eat or bathe.

If you have a strong support system at home, the decision to have a procedure is that much easier, and so is recovery. If you don't have strong support, let your physician know.

THE TYPICAL COSTS OF FACIAL REJUVENATION

- **Skin-care products:** $75–$200 per month
- **Botox:** $250–$800 per treatment (depends on the area; typically $16–$20 per unit: 15–20 units for crow's feet, 15–25 units for frown lines, 10–20 units for forehead lines; men need more units than women)
- **Restylane, Juvéderm, Perlane:** $550–$650 per syringe (typically need 2–3 syringes for face, 1–2 syringes for lips)
- **Radiesse:** $800–$900 per syringe (typically need 2–3 syringes)
- **Sculptra:** $1,250–$1,500 per vial (3–4 vials average per person)
- **Rhinoplasty:** $9,000–$20,000 (depending on complexity)
- **Forehead lift:** $7,500–$12,000
- **Blepharoplasty:** $3,500–$8,000
- **Fat grafting:** $6,500–$9,000
- **Face-lift:** $12,000–$25,000
- **Fractional laser:** $1,000 per treatment (typically need 3–4 treatments)
- **CO_2 laser:** $4,000

Question 10: Am I Really Ready for the Thing I Think I Want?

This is not simple question, but it's a great one to end our quiz. Being ready is different from being able to afford the procedure or take the time off to recover (as we alluded to in question 8). Being ready means being prepared physically *and* mentally; both have to work in concert for you to get the best results.

Frankly, some people just aren't ready. They waffle about what they want, not because they don't know but because subconsciously they realize that they're not ready to have anything done just yet.

We can usually spot this fairly early, but convincing the patient is another story. That's why asking yourself now, before you have anything done, is so important.

The Consultation: Expectations, Questions, and Answers

We are not in a cookie-cutter business. The beauty of faces is that no two are exactly alike. Even identical twins—who may start out with startlingly similar features—will develop unique and personal differences throughout their lives. Many variables—a beard, a way of applying makeup, five or ten additional or fewer pounds—can affect one's appearance.

Likewise, the aging process affects every individual differently. Genetic, environmental, and gravitational forces have a significant impact on facial appearance. A comprehensive facial rejuvenation consultation should discuss skin care, noninvasive procedures, and surgical management in a way that is tailored to each individual patient. A systematic approach must be undertaken to address the face, eyes, nose, and neck in their entirety in order to obtain a balanced, natural, and "unoperated" appearance. We recommend a four-part consultation for maximum benefits.

Part 1: Preventive Measures

Many people want absolute answers and black-and-white results, but neither life nor medicine works that way. Any procedure we undertake depends on our skill and your participation, so be an active participant. You also need to be realistic; beauty is a process, not a procedure.

Accordingly, the first part of the consultation should focus on preventive measures to slow down the aging process. The following considerations will be discussed:

- Anti-aging regimen
- Skin-care consultation with a professional aesthetician
- Sun-protection regimen
- Tobacco cessation
- Image consultation
- Dietary changes

Part 2: Noninvasive Procedures

The second phase of the consultation should address noninvasive procedures to improve facial appearance. Many people will not need any surgical intervention. The options include the following:

- Laser resurfacing
- Chemical peels
- Soft-tissue augmentation and fillers: Restylane, Juvéderm, Perlane, Evolence, Radiesse, Sculptra
- BOTOX Cosmetic
- Fat grafting
- Thermage, Titan

Part 3: Surgery Specifics

The third aspect of the consultation should be designed to discuss areas of the face that will benefit from facial plastic surgery. All regions of the face must be evaluated in order to achieve a balanced and aesthetically pleasing outcome. When applicable, surgical and nonsurgical methods are often combined in order to get the optimum outcome; we call these *complementary proce-dures*, and we will discuss them at length in future chapters. The following regions and surgical options are typically discussed in a thorough and realistic consultation:

The brow-eye complex
- Blepharoplasty (plastic surgery of the eyelids)
- Brow lift (endoscopic forehead lift)
- Fat grafting

The midface and nasolabial fold region
- Face-lift (rhytidectomy)
- Endoscopic midface-lift

AGE IS JUST A NUMBER

We are big advocates of beauty at any age, so it's hard for us to say no because of a chronological number. We see people as young as their early teens, and sometimes even preteens or "tweens," to fix scars, remove growths, enhance the appearance of a nose, or correct ear deformities.

Particularly in Hollywood, where parents are willing to invest thousands of dollars to help turn their son or daughter into the next child star, facial rejuvenation patients are getting younger and younger. We're not alone in seeing this phenomenon: according to the American Society of Plastic Surgeons, "over 333,000 people 18 years and younger had plastic surgery in 2005, up from about 306,000 in 2000."

Of course, beauty isn't the only reason for a young person to have plastic surgery. How about the young child who's been in an accident, who was born with facial paralysis, who suffered a vicious attack by the neighborhood stray dog, or who disfigured his or her face in a fireworks or household accident? These cases require special care, and we usually want the children to have surgery when they are younger rather than older, to avail themselves of the recuperative properties of young skin and to avoid being teased in their tough social environment.

At the opposite end of the age spectrum, we've had patients as old as their early eighties come in looking for the rejuvenation that

- Cheek implants (malar and submalar)
- Multilevel fat grafting
- Rhinoplasty (nasal reshaping, nose job)

The lower face and neck
- Face-lift and neck lift (rhytidectomy)
- Chin augmentation
- Fat grafting

An *endoscope* is a specially designed telescope that allows your surgeon to do precise surgical work through a tiny incision inside the hairline in order to avoid scarring in the more sensitive facial areas. The forehead and the midface (cheek) are the

is reserved mostly for people in their fifties and sixties. One of us (Dr. Hamilton) had a great-aunt who had a face-lift at eighty-two years old and lived to be ninety-nine! Just as with patients who are too young, however, we must also be careful with patients who might be too old to endure invasive surgical procedures.

With both the young and the old, however, each individual is different, and not everyone comes to us merely for beautification— even in Beverly Hills!

We have created a system called an Aging Arc in order to describe a person's "visual" age versus his or her actual chronological age. Our goal in aesthetic medicine is to put our patients in the positive range on the Aging Arc, which means that they appear radiant and the best they can for their age. People in the negative range appear either older than their chronological age or drastically younger due to cosmetic intervention.

Although environmental factors can have irreversible outcomes, facial rejuvenation techniques can prolong one's position in the positive range of the Aging Arc. Anti-aging methods and appearing younger do not involve a complete overhaul of appearance. Minor tweaks, which may be unnoticeable to the untrained eye, can create an overall youthful effect on one's appearance. People should not strive to be unnaturally young-looking, because ultimately, the excessive surgical procedures that that requires will negatively alter the way one looks.

most common areas that can be addressed using the endoscope. The lower face (jowls) and the neck are not typically treated with the endoscope.

Part 4: Aftercare

The final phase of the consultation process should involve professional makeup artists and hairstylists to enhance and optimize the results that have been achieved through noninvasive and surgical methods. After all, you want to maintain and enhance the results, don't you? Take pains to learn as much as you can about the beautification process in this all-important step.

Camouflage techniques for the initial healing process should be discussed in order to allow the patient to return to normal daily activities as soon as possible. (A skin-care regimen with professional consultation should be continued.)

The following aftercare should be discussed:

- Image consultants
- Hairstylists
- Makeup artists
- Anti-aging regimen
- Skin-care regimen and consultation
- Dietary changes

A face-lift alone cannot be considered a complete facial rejuvenation. A comprehensive approach must be utilized to obtain consistent, natural, and long-lasting results.

What Is Your Current Medical Condition?

It is important to remember that even nonsurgical procedures can introduce a host of chemicals into your skin and therefore your body. To best know how to treat you—and which treatments to possibly avoid—your physician must know your current physical condition and any drugs or medications that you are taking.

Have you been depressed lately? Did you become out of breath walking from the parking lot to the doctor's office? Are you a smoker? Believe it or not, these are all critical issues your doctor must explore before, during, and after the consultation, so be honest and forthcoming. Your health could depend on it!

The following medical issues should be discussed during the consultation:

- Smoking
- Thyroid
- Dry eye syndrome
- Depression
- Cardiac disease
- Kidney and liver disease
- Herpes
- Weight and body mass index (BMI)
- Medications
- Autoimmune diseases, such as lupus

3

Face Value

Answers by Areas

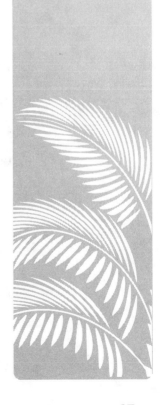

Faces, like fingerprints, are unique to each and every one of us. Some of us have fair complexions, others are swarthy. Whereas one has "apples" in his cheeks, another has finely chiseled cheekbones. Some of us have fine, delicate features; others have big, broad features. Some have oily skin, and some have dry skin. Which of these describes you?

The answer might surprise you. In our practices, we find that many people are often unfamiliar with their own faces. Strange as it may seem, the more they look at their faces in the mirror, the less they recognize them as their own. People often have difficulty evaluating their faces objectively.

What often appears most disfiguring to others, from an unattractive mole to a pronounced area of facial aging, may be overlooked by the people who have it. Sometimes this can be explained by long duration (you've always had it, so you don't notice it) versus recent onset (you never had it before, so you really notice it). A common example with no ready explanation is that minimal upper-lip lines drive some women crazy, but these same women overlook their more noticeable brow droop or cheek laxity. Many times the most recent change takes precedence over the root problem.

In fact, many individuals are under false assumptions about the definition of *beauty*, and some are even viewing their faces through the lenses of negative self-talk that has often taken years to create. For example, suppose a young girl hears one or two negative phrases associated with her nose or some other so-called prominent feature. Maybe it's something innocuous, like her little brother calling her "big nose" during a fight or a visiting relative opining, "My, what big ears you have!" Over time, these statements can become exaggerated in the child's mind until they are almost grandiose. Add to these complaints the typical rigors of the aging process—with its inherent changes in complexion, skin tone, and facial features as well as sagging and wrinkles—and the patient's negative self-talk can reach a critical mass—the point at which she believes that *something* must be done.

At other times the complaints people have are entirely their own—without any objective input whatsoever. One patient hates her "fleshy face." Another can't stand his "sagging eyelids." She hates her crow's feet, and he wishes he had more heft to his chin. Again, over time, these complaints become extremely important.

As a result, you know *what* you see (or what you think you see), but not *why* you see it. Whatever your complaint about your face may be, it's valid—at least, to you. We are not here to judge or pressure you into feeling great about your face or bad about your face; it's your face, after all. Our only job is to provide the necessary objectivity so that you can make educated, sound decisions about surgical or nonsurgical procedures on and around the face.

It is important to recognize that not everything can be corrected. Genetics play as big a role in the aging and development process as your behavior does. It is the combination of the two that makes us who we are, unique individuals with our own definitions of beauty.

In this chapter, we discuss the major areas of the face from top to bottom, starting with the forehead and brows and extending all the way down to the neck. Along the way we discuss the effects of aging, how those unique features of yours might be detracting from your overall "look," and, for each facial area, the pros and cons of current procedures.

As you read, we suggest that you keep a mirror handy. The handheld kind works best; it's light and portable, so you can pick it up and put it down at will. This way, when we discuss specific terms like *crepey* or *brittle*, you can quickly do a spot-check to see how you measure up. As we mentioned earlier in this book, you must be a partner with your physician, matching him or her step for step when it comes to knowing your own face and asking the right questions.

In our practices, we have found that the most successful individuals are those who come to us well informed, free of emotion, and open to discussion. By reading this chapter thoroughly, exploring your own features in the mirror along the way, and keeping an open mind, you will be more familiar with your face by the end of this chapter than you ever thought you would be.

When It Comes to Aging, Your Face Is on the Front Lines

Aging is a natural occurrence; it happens to everybody. You can neither avoid it nor, despite what the makers of various creams and potions may claim, entirely prevent it. Of course, we all age differently. Some women have gray hair in their thirties, whereas others don't have it until their sixties. Some men keep their youthful, fit physique well into their seventies, whereas others lose it in their early forties.

Genetics play a part, to be sure, but so does behavior. Daily exercise and proper nutrition can help us to maintain stronger and leaner bodies at any age, well into our eighties. Yet good behavior can do only so much; if your hair is meant (because of your genes) to become gray when you're thirty, you'd better learn to love it or find an affordable colorist in your neighborhood.

When it comes to genetics, we must play the hand we've been dealt. If your DNA is hardwired to make you stop growing at five feet six inches, there is very little you can do about that. Likewise, your skin has genetic traits that cause it to age in a particular manner at certain stages and at certain ages. The effects of aging can begin as early as your twenties. This is when various blemishes, wrinkles, and even sun-induced spots begin to appear and become part of your facial makeup.

As we age, our face loses elasticity, or flexibility. In addition, our facial bone structure changes as we lose both density and mass. We also lose collagen, a protein complex in the skin that binds the area together to keep a youthful, firm structure. Volume loss, which contributes to the hollow look we often see in the faces of aging individuals, is a critical factor. Bone loss in the upper and lower jaws and loss of facial fat inevitably lead to smile and marionette furrows, laxity of the cheeks, and eyelid hollows.

Again, these are forces of nature; they happen to us all. Each decade brings with it many more noticeable changes. You can see this by viewing photographs of yourself through the years; line them up chronologically and you can see in living color how age has affected your face.

What about our behavior, however? How can what we do affect how we look? You'd be surprised how behaviors such as excessive sun exposure, smoking, and even undereating can affect how your face ages. According to the American Academy of Dermatology, "Too much sun can cause sunburn, wrinkles, freckles, skin texture changes, dilated blood vessels, and skin cancers."

According to Mayo Clinic dermatologist Dr. Lawrence Gibson, "Smoking causes narrowing of the blood vessels in the outermost layers of your skin. This impairs blood flow to your skin, depleting it of oxygen and important nutrients, such as vitamin A." The result is a decrease in elasticity and an increase in wrinkles.

Undereating can make our faces too thin. We all need a certain amount of fullness in the face; that might not be the most scientific term to describe it, but it's certainly a proper way to describe cheeks that are sufficiently full, if not plump, and skin that is elastic, healthy, and less likely to wrinkle. Think of a balloon; when it is full, it is taut and wrinkle-free. As the air slowly leaks out, the balloon thins and begins to wrinkle and sag. The effects on the face are generally the same.

That is why doctors talk about "baby fat"—that vibrant, firm fullness of youth—in positive terms, even though most of our patients speak of it in negative terms. When they see their faces as "fat" or "fleshy," we know the dangers of aging to come, and we recognize that a full, firm face now can actually serve them well in the future.

The aging process revolves around four critical factors:

1. **Rhytids—wrinkles (skin ages and loses elasticity).** If you've ever spent an afternoon playing pickup basketball with your younger relatives on a holiday weekend—particularly if you're not used to doing so on a daily or even weekly basis—you will know that your muscles don't quite "bounce back" the way they used to when you were a teenager. Your skin is much the same. Skin consistency changes as we age, so we end up with fine lines, aging spots, and an entirely different skin texture. We lose the "snap" factor: the skin's ability to snap back into place if you pinch, press, pound, or pull it. Try it now, with your mirror. Pinch a spot on your cheek or neck and time how long it takes to snap back into place; the older you are, the slower this will be. Now try the experiment on a teenager or an older relative (if anyone will let you!). The differences can be amazing.

2. **Furrows—dynamic muscle contraction.** You contort your facial muscles into a variety of expressions—sad, puzzled, fearful, happy, angry—and they all take a toll eventually.

Despite their advantage to you in conveying emotions, these muscle movements also cause aging furrows (*expression lines*). Specifically, they form on the forehead, around the eyes, and around the mouth. When you're younger, these lines come and go with your expression; as you age, they become more permanently etched into your face. That is, when you're younger, smile lines or crow's feet appear only while you're smiling or squinting, respectively; when you're older, the lines remain even after the expression on your face is long gone. Loss of skin elasticity tends to increase the depth and persistence of these expression lines. Didn't your mother ever tell you, "Be careful; your face will freeze like that"? Well, she might not have been so wrong after all.

3. **Laxity.** You may not know what *laxity* means yet, but you will know it when you see it: it is looseness and sagginess. This has to do with the effects of gravity and aging on skin. Individuals who have weak bone structure (small chins and cheekbones) don't have good support for soft tissue, so they tend to have more laxity—and at an earlier age.

4. **Facial atrophy—volume loss.** As the face naturally loses its fullness, or volume, over the years, it becomes less supple and more brittle. There is less wiggle room, so to speak, when it comes to handling facial expressions and other environmental factors such as exposure to the sun or smoking. Not only is the skin sagging, as many people tend to claim, it's also losing the fullness and suppleness of its younger years. We can compare the face of a younger person to a grape and the face of an older person to a raisin; this is the result of volume loss. Several contributing factors to volume loss include the following:

   - Less fat in the face as we age
   - Bone, cartilage, and facial structure changes that affect the chin, nose, jaws, and brows. Think about individuals who have dentures or poor dental hygiene. Their faces look significantly older. That is because poor dental health leads to significant bone loss in the upper and lower jaws.
   - Loss of muscle volume over time

The Effects of Aging—There Goes the Neighborhood

The key to aging gracefully is to look at the face as a whole. That brings us to the notion of "the neighborhood." The different parts of your face blend together to form one larger body: a whole, the neighborhood. Every neighborhood, like every face, is unique; some houses are big, some houses are small. Some neighborhoods themselves are large and complex; others are small and compact.

Just as you can drive through a neighborhood and get a certain feel for the residents and how they care for their vicinity, so too do faces have a certain look or feel, based on the sum of their parts. The sum would be quite different if the parts were not so unique. In other words, if you change your nose, you don't fix just one house on the block; the whole neighborhood looks different as a result.

As doctors, we are forced to look at the pieces as pieces and the sum as the sum; it is in our job descriptions. Yet we are also forced to take into consideration exactly how those pieces relate to the sum, how the parts form the whole. It would be irresponsible of us to make one change that we know would result in a less appealing result; we try to explain this to our patients, and we will try to explain it to you, our readers.

We often try to provide a resolution that relies on two avenues: surgical and nonsurgical. Not only are some procedures better for certain individuals, ages, or parts of the face, some combinations of surgical and nonsurgical procedures are also better than, for instance, a surgical procedure alone.

In other words, there is no easy answer to what (you think) ails you. The face, like beauty itself, is a complex neighborhood of large points and small, broad strokes and fine. We must work together as doctor and patient to understand what combination of effects you are looking for and how to create them.

In the rest of this chapter, we discuss the major areas of the face as follows, so that you can better assess your own needs:

- Forehead and brows (upper face)
- Eyes
- Cheeks (midface)
- Nose
- Mouth
- Jawline and chin (lower face)
- Neck

Before our analysis of particular facial areas begins, we survey the face as a whole, noting skin texture, discoloration, and blemishes. Skin can have a significant impact on your whole face.

Bad skin is like a sad, cloudy day in the neighborhood, whereas great skin is like a sunny day—fresh, airy, and light. The shape of the face and the positions of the facial features also have to be analyzed for any major discrepancy. This survey provides an overview that allows us to have a much better idea of a patient's entire appearance.

The Forehead and the Brows

We start our tour of the facial neighborhood at the top, with your forehead and brows. How these two regions work together—and separately—is a great example of why we treat the face as a whole rather than as a collection of unrelated parts. The forehead is actually lifting the eyebrows so that you can see better. We sometimes refer to this as the "height of facial expression" because it is both literally the highest part of expression and symbolically where your expression begins.

If you could avoid all facial expression, you could retain a much more youthful appearance well into old age. Studies have been done on schizophrenics—who do not express emotion the way the rest of us do and so have a limited number of facial expressions—and they have been found to have a much more youthful appearance, and for longer, than their more normal counterparts. We certainly don't recommend avoiding facial expressions, but this example shows how facial expressions do affect the face in the form of lines and wrinkles.

Your forehead is integral to each and every facial movement you make, even blinking or winking. Look in the mirror. See how the broad expanse of your forehead tends to wrinkle or bunch with the slightest movement? Do people think you're angry when you're not?

Naturally, over time, the lines in the forehead will deepen and become permanent. What quickly snapped back in youth now takes longer and longer to ease back into shape. Eventually, those wrinkles become the shape of the forehead and the brow, and this is one of the main reasons that both men and women of a certain age come to see us.

Common issues with the brows and the forehead include the following:

- Lines between the brows ("eleven sign")
- Forehead lines
- Brow ptosis, or drooping brows

The most common complaint about the brow and forehead region is nagging lines across the forehead and between the eyebrows. We refer to the latter as the "eleven (11) sign," for obvious reasons.

In the "before" photo below, the furrow between the brows looks like the number 11. This is an expression feature that

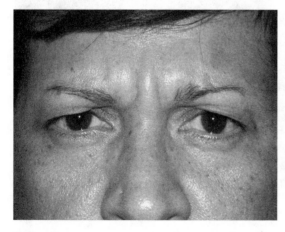

Before Botox

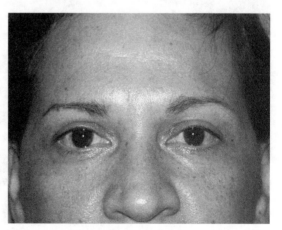

After Botox and blepharoplasty

evolves over time from the contracting of the facial muscles when you show concern, worry, doubt, or apprehension. The loss of elasticity in the skin will leave this permanent furrow between your brows, and it will require some type of medical attention if you are concerned enough about it to seek a remedy.

The right-hand figure on page 45 shows the effects of Botox on a furrowed brow. (Note: This person has also had blepharoplasty, or an eyelid lift.) In later chapters we will discuss the various surgical and nonsurgical options involved in erasing these lines.

The second most common complaint about the forehead is "My eyebrows are sagging." As doctors, we have to qualify that statement. Sagging skin, as we have seen, is the result of a variety of factors. We call the sagging of eyebrows *brow ptosis*.

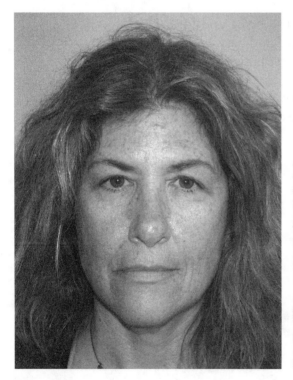

Brow ptosis

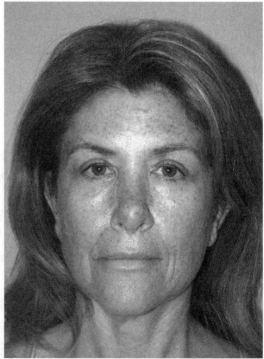

After endoscopic brow lift and blepharoplasty

Sometimes it is due to age, but often it is genetic, with the problem beginning in youth. Brow ptosis typically occurs on the outer portion or tail of the eyebrows.

The Eyes

We know that the aging changes around the eyes do not just involve sagging skin. There are multiple components, such as loss of skin elasticity, drooping and deflation of the eyebrows and cheek pads, and weakness of the supporting eyelid structures, which leads to puffiness under the eyes. The forehead and cheeks also should be thoroughly evaluated. Common aging changes around the eyes include the following:

- Lines around the eyes, or crow's feet
- Laxity and bags under the eyes
- Skin hanging above the eyes, or droopy eyelids

In the neighborhood of your face, we consider your brow to be the "upstairs neighbor" of your eyes. By the eyes, we mean not only the lids of the eyes but also the shape and circumference of the eyes themselves, as well as the surrounding tissues and features. Like many upstairs neighbors, the brow is not always so considerate of its downstairs neighbor! In fact, as we just saw in the previous section, the brow is often "knocking on the door" and causing trouble for your eyes.

Much as the eyes' upstairs neighbor isn't always a good one to have, their "downstairs neighbors"—otherwise known as the cheeks—also affect the quality, size, and shape of your eyes. As you age and the cheeks experience volume loss, they almost tend to deflate.

Naturally, as pressure from the brow above and volume loss from the cheeks below converge in the eye region, the entire neighborhood of the face is affected. Common complaints from individuals include drooping above the eyes and wrinkling and pinching below and in the corners of the eyes. The photos on pages 46 and 48 show a variety of ways in which the eyes can age and be repaired.

Before upper
blepharoplasty

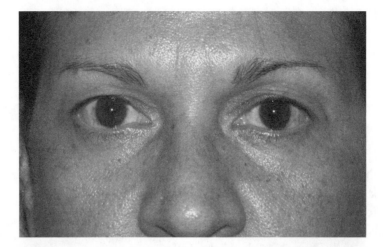

After upper
blepharoplasty,
without makeup

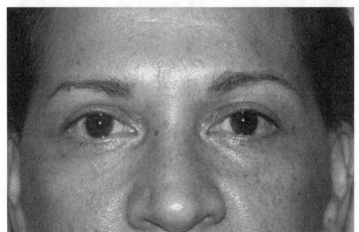

After upper
blepharoplasty,
with makeup

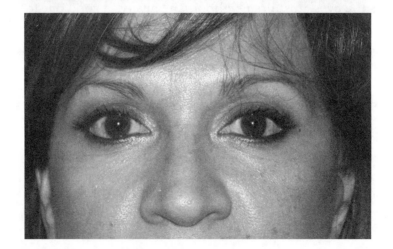

As skin elasticity decreases, you see shadows, depressions, and cavities around the eyes; these are hallmarks of the aging process. It is our job to see that whichever procedure we and our patients decide on together, we not only make improvements on the eye features themselves but also create features that are harmonious with the rest of the face. This often involves addressing brow and cheek concerns as well as the eye concerns that the person has.

The Cheeks

Your cheeks—and their underlying bone structure—can often be likened to the walls of the "house" (your face). You don't hear as much about cheeks as you do about brows, eyes, and chins, but in fact the loss of volume in the cheek area has a ripple effect throughout the face that affects all of the above.

Some common issues relating to the cheeks include the following:

- Hollows and depressions
- Sagging cheeks
- Prominent nasolabial folds

As you can see in the illustration on page 50, the cheeks—or the midface, as this area is called by aesthetic professionals—are integral to your facial makeup.

One simple way in which we like to think and talk about cheeks is to remind people that an aged appearance is flat, whereas youthfulness is round. In other words, what captivates and inspires us about youth is its full, round, vibrant features, with lots of highlights. During the aging process, the midface starts to flatten out, and slight hollows and depressions start to appear, causing shadows rather than highlights.

As a quick homework assignment, put down this book and revisit some photos of yourself. Compare the pictures from when you were in your twenties and thirties to pictures of yourself in your fifties and sixties. (If you are not this old, use photos of an older family member.) In the more youthful pictures, you will often see a prevailing theme of lots of highlights: smiling

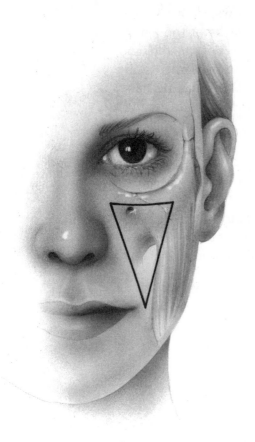

The midface area

expressions, fullness of face, and no sharpness or harshness reflecting back at you.

In the pictures of you in your fifties or sixties, you can begin to notice more sharpness in the features as the effects of aging take place; typically, this is the result of a loss of volume and fullness. You might see lots of shadows in these pictures.

The most common reason that people come see us about their cheeks is the deepening of "laugh lines," or nasolabial folds. Many come because, quite frankly, they're unhappy with either sagging cheeks or a tired, gaunt look.

The effects of aging—the loss of volume and the deterioration of bone and shape—have left these people feeling undistinguished. In such cases they often want more cheek fullness and less prominence of nasolabial folds. These issues can be resolved surgically through fat transfer or nonsurgically through fillers (both of which we will discuss in later chapters).

A more disturbing trend we've been seeing recently is young people who want to get rid of their facial baby fat by removing the *buccal fat pad*. We are very careful to tell them that the buccal fat pad is important not just to the look of a healthy face but to the actual health of an aging face.

We've spoken frequently about the loss of volume and its effects on the face as we age. Taking the buccal fat pad from a youthful, rounded face is like jump-starting a volume-loss chain reaction: the more you take away in youth, the less that will be present as you age. In fact, one very common treatment for bolstering cheeks and cheekbone structure is to inject fat into the face to create a more defined and distinguished look in a cheek structure that has suffered from lack of volume. Thus, you can actually accelerate the aging process by taking out the buccal fat pads that cause baby fat.

People often believe that there is a timeline of facial aging therapy, starting with various noninvasive procedures like skin-care products, microdermabrasion, and fillers and extending to surgical procedures such as midface-lifts and fat grafting. The reality is that there is not one timeline: these noninvasive and surgical procedures often treat quite different problems. It's more like multiple timelines, each with different treatments. Some things need help early, others later.

Let's talk a little about how surgical and nonsurgical procedures work together. For instance, many people think that a face-lift solves all the major problems associated with the facial "neighborhood": the forehead, brows, eyelids, eyes, cheeks, jaw, and chin. However, this would be like saying that a tune-up makes your car 100 percent ready for the road; it doesn't. What if there isn't enough air in the tires? What if the tires aren't aligned? What if you still need an oil change?

Likewise, a face-lift is the right procedure at the right time for the right reasons—but not for all people all the time for all reasons. We often see people with already thin faces who want a face-lift to accentuate their cheeks and give their bone structure more definition. A generic face-lift would pull an already hollow face even tighter, creating a flatter, aging effect rather than a more rounded, youthful effect.

For a patient who wants a face-lift but really needs fat grafting or nonsurgical injectables, first we educate her about why a face-lift isn't in her best interest, then we show her some "before" and "after" pictures that illustrate our recommendations, and finally, we suggest an alternate plan that's right for her.

The right solution for your particular problem might be a little surgery, some nonsurgical options, and some lifestyle changes. For instance, when people have a lean body mass, they tend to lose fat in the cheeks, so it's very hard to both stay slim and age well.

Thus, there are things that you can actively do to prevent the fat loss that contributes to the hollow look that often comes with aging. As you can see, facial augmentation is a partnership between doctor and patient—in more ways than one.

The Nose

The nose plays a central role in the neighborhood. It occupies the center of the face; therefore, any major outstanding features it has will be a distraction from the eyes, which should always be the focus of the face. A very large nose, for example, can be the "elephant in the room"—the thing that everyone sees but no one talks about. The nose can also play a very prominent role in a person's profile in conjunction with the chin. The nose should fit the face, the body, and the ethnicity of an individual. For instance, Asian individuals with overly Westernized noses will lose their ethnic looks and their charm and appeal.

The nose is composed of bone and cartilage covered by a thin layer of fat and skin. The upper portion of the nose is bone, whereas the middle and lower segments are composed of three-dimensional cartilage. The nasal cartilages are the foundation of the nose. Internally, the septum divides the nasal passageway into two distinct compartments—it's like the center divider of a busy two-way highway. Deviation of the septum is the main cause of breathing difficulty. Think about what happens when there is an accident on one side of the freeway.

Most of our rhinoplasty (nose job) patients have had life-long concerns about the appearance of their noses. However, rhinoplasty has also become a major part of facial rejuvenation during the aging process, because the nose undergoes significant changes at that time. The skin over the bone and cartilage thins out and loses elasticity, while the cartilage starts to separate from the bony structure, causing the nose to elongate and droop.

We typically analyze the bridge and tip of the nose from a front view and a profile view in order to understand the issues that are causing concern to the individuals. From the frontal view, the bridge of the nose should have a straight appearance, without significant crookedness. There are shad-

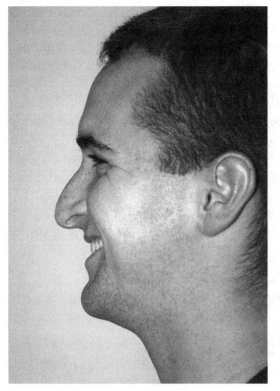

Before rhinoplasty

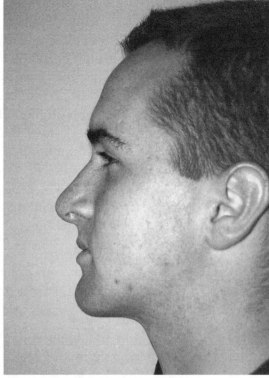

After rhinoplasty

ows that should follow the inner aspect of the brow down to the tip. The tip should have soft shadows without significantly sharp edges. The nasal tip must not be too thin or too bulbous. From the profile, we first analyze the relationship of the nose and chin.

A person with a recessed small chin (a condition known as *microgenia*) can appear to have a large nose, and vice versa. After the profile has been thoroughly analyzed, we turn our attention to the bridge of the nose. A large hump or, conversely, a shallow bridge (called *saddle nose deformity*) brings unwanted attention to the nose. Furthermore, the relationship of the bridge as it leads into the tip should be gentle and smooth. The projection of the tip away from the face and its relationship to the upper lip should also be carefully analyzed.

The Mouth

When people say "mouth," in reference to facial rejuvenation, they usually mean the lips. They could be referring to the fullness of the lips, the thinness of the lips, the shape of the lips, or even the color or texture of the lips.

The changing texture of the skin as it ages creates deepening lines above, below, and around the lips. These are often the result of years of smoking, or they can merely be a sign of age and lost elasticity in the skin due to sun exposure and/or repeated facial expressions. The latter is a much more important contributing factor for women, for some reason.

The major complaints about the mouth region are as follows:

- Thin lips
- Lines around the mouth ("smoker's lines")
- Lines from the corner of the mouth to chin ("marionette lines")

In later chapters, we discuss a variety of options to help define and accentuate lips that are too thin. Again, the goal is to give you what you need rather than what you think you want. We've all seen lips that go from too thin to too big, so our job is to give you lips that are just right.

Lines around the lips, which are often called smoker's lines even when they are not associated with smoking, present another set of problems. These are usually solved through the use of various nonsurgical fillers, peels, and/or laser applications.

"Marionette lines," which extend from the corners of the mouth to the chin, are often the most telltale sign of aging. These lines are caused by bone loss in the area along with shifting tissue. Fillers, fat grafting, and/or chin implants can correct them very effectively.

The Jawline and the Chin

As we near the end of our tour of the neighborhood that is our unique, individual face, we come to the lower face: the jawline and the chin. Here, in essence, is the very foundation of the face.

If the brow is the roof and the cheeks are the walls of our facial structure, then the jaw line and the chin define the ground floor, or foundation, of the face.

Common lower-face issues include the following:

- Sagging jowls
- Weak chin
- Volume loss

We see people complaining about their jowls on a weekly basis. Gravity is the main culprit in creating jowls, for both men and women. You can almost feel the earth tugging down on the skin and resulting in the sagging that creates jowls.

Although a host of both surgical and nonsurgical remedies are available for this situation, it is important to be realistic about the potential results and to be an active participant in understanding the challenges that are involved in achieving those results.

Some individuals are less concerned with the jowls themselves and are more interested in creating a stronger jawline. Once again, even though this is a mostly surgical procedure, it is important to keep in mind how changing one aspect of the face affects all the other areas.

The other main complaint about the lower face is a weak chin. The photographs on page 56 show how a face-lift in combination with chin augmentation can remedy this.

A chin is not just a chin; it is part of an entire face. Unlike the cheeks, which are more flesh and less bone, the chin is less flesh and more bone. Shape and density are also concerns. A strong profile requires a strong chin. How does the shape of the jaw affect the chin, and vice versa? The chin-to-nose relationship is important, too, because the size of the chin affects our perception of the nose: a small chin equals a large nose.

Other questions we must ask are as follows: How old is the patient? In what condition are his or her teeth? Teeth play a large role in shaping the chin, in angle and density as well as in the smile and "marionette lines." Poor dentition usually leads to erosion of the jaw bone, which is also known as the mandible. We often recommend working in concert with a patient's dentist

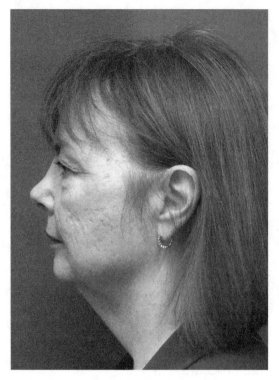
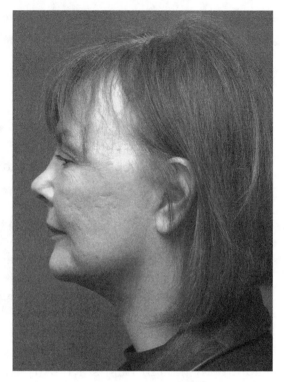

Before facial, neck, and eyelid rejuvenation   After facial, neck, and eyelid rejuvenation

to create a beautiful smile and teeth that complement the rest of the face.

Although the jowls can occasionally be addressed with non-surgical procedures, surgical face-lifts give the best long-term outcome for moderate to advanced jowls. The chin region is just as frequently rectified with surgical means like chin implants or fat grafting. This is a serious decision that will affect the rest of the face.

These are all issues to discuss with your doctor, one-to-one. We recommend that you highlight the passages in this book that interest you, concern you, alarm you, and even confuse you; then take the book to your facial plastic surgeon or dermatologist and discuss these passages with him or her. If your doctor can address your concerns in a way that makes you feel more comfortable, then all of us have done our jobs.

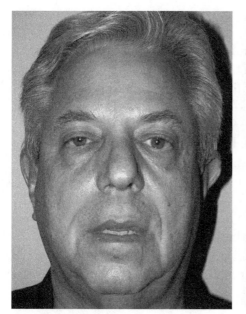

Before surgery, front view

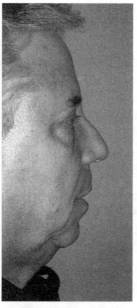

Before surgery, profile view

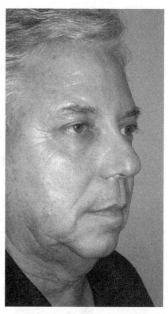

Before surgery, quarter view

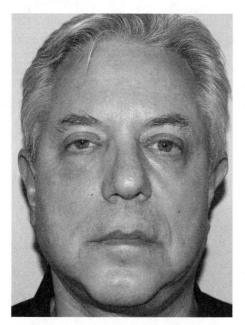

After face-lift and chin augmentation, front view

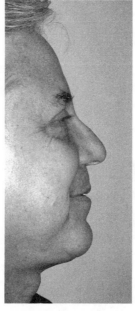

After face-lift and chin augmentation, profile view

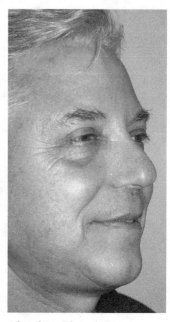

After face-lift and chin augmentation, quarter view

The Neck

The neck is a particularly vulnerable section of the facial neighborhood. Aging really takes a toll on the neck, for it is to here that skin often heads as gravity pulls it down along and even past the face, creating a "turkey neck" look that brings many a patient into our offices.

There are two parts of the body where it is very hard to hide the aging process: the neck and the hands. These are highly visible and sensitive parts of the body.

When analyzing your neck, you should take into account the relationship between the chin and the internal bones above your voice box. The sharpness of the neck depends on the position of these structures. One of the first questions we like to ask people who are unhappy with the appearance of the neck is "Have you ever liked your neck?" The reason we ask this question is

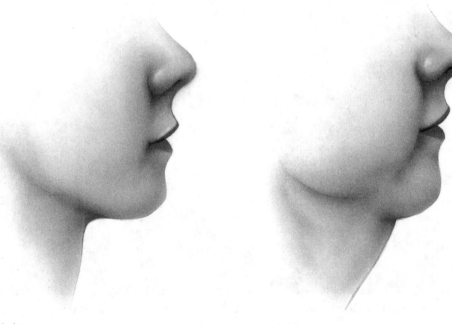

A youthful chin   An aged chin

HOW WE FIX FACIAL PROBLEMS

	Problem	Solution
Forehead and brows	Forehead lines and lines between brows	Botox/fillers
	Drooping brows	Endoscopic brow lift/ fat grafting
Eyes	Sagging eyelids	Blepharoplasty
	Bags under eyes	Fat grafting/blepharoplasty
	Crow's feet	Botox
	Fine lines	Chemical peels Lasers
Cheeks	Nasolabial folds ("laugh lines") and hollows	Fillers/fat grafting/ midface implants
	Sagging cheeks	Endoscopic midface-lift
Nose	Prominent profile or tip	Rhinoplasty
Mouth	"Smoker's lines"	Fillers, Botox, lasers
	"Marionette lines"	
	Thin lips	
Jaw and chin	Jowls	Face-lift (with or without fillers and/or fat)
	Weak chin	Chin augmentation (implants or fillers)
Neck	Neck bands	Botox, Face-lift/neck lift
	Neck fat	Liposuction

that many patients have unfavorable anatomy that leads to very premature aging of the neck. For instance, if you have a weak chin, the neck tends to look nonexistent.

During the aging process of the neck, the skin becomes loose, fat can accumulate under the neck, and the muscles of the neck (platysma) can weaken and separate, resulting in "neck bands." The illustrations on page 58 show how the neck looks during the typical aging process—and what hope lies through a variety of available procedures.

What You Can Do Today to Spruce Up the Neighborhood: Three Tips for an Age-Proof Face

There you have it: our grand tour of the neighborhood that is your face. From forehead to neck, we have not only seen how aging affects the face but have also caught a glimpse of how a variety of surgical and nonsurgical applications can remedy your facial concerns.

There are positive, proactive things that each person can do to influence the way he or she ages. In later chapters we will discuss nonsurgical and surgical solutions to the most common problems. To conclude this chapter, we offer the following three foolproof tips for how, starting today, to prevent some of the effects of aging on the face:

- **Less sun, more sunscreen.** Stop worshiping the sun and start caring for your skin instead. We can't say this enough. We all enjoy a day at the beach and the fresh, attractive feeling we have when our faces are suntanned—or sunburned. However, spending too much time in the sun is like squandering your savings account in your youth only to regret it in your golden years—you will pay for it later. We've seen how the sun damages the skin; avoid harmful ultraviolet (UV) rays when you can and protect yourself from them when you can't. It's as simple as that. Use a total (UVB and UVA) sunblock (see the next chapter for exact recommendations).
- **Quit smoking.** If you're still smoking, quit. If you're thinking about starting to smoke, don't. If your coworkers smoke, avoid them—or get them to quit. The chemicals and heat from a burning cigarette wreak obvious havoc on your face, and it isn't always easy to remove. If you want to start achieving a more youthful appearance tomorrow, quit smoking today. Nicotine has been shown in numerous laboratory experiments to harm the various components of the dermis (a deeper layer of the skin).

- **Stop worrying.** What's done is done; you can't go back in time. If you were a sun worshiper in your youth or smoked until just yesterday, quit crying over spilled milk; it won't do any good. All you can do is move on from today and look forward to tomorrow. You can quit adding to the lines that are already etched into your face by worrying less from this day forward. Revel in the knowledge that modern techniques can delay or reverse the effects of aging.

4

Lotions and Potions

How to Prevent or Reverse the Aging Process

God hath given you one face, and you make yourselves another.

—WILLIAM SHAKESPEARE

Wouldn't it be great if we could turn back time? How much more confident would you feel if you could act as you do today, in midlife, yet have the wrinkle-free, firm, and elastic skin tone of your twenties or even your thirties? What a great combination that would be: wisdom *and* beauty, experience *and* exfoliation!

It's the age-old "If I had only known then what I know now" dilemma, and modern science is helping you to make it a reality with each passing day. Skin creams, ampoules, treatments, lotions, and potions are all the rage—and with good reason: we are a nation obsessed with youth, worshiping at its altar and coming away feeling worse about our older, smarter selves.

It's no secret that the popular media, funded by advertising dollars from the world's top corporations, feed this youth-oriented craze like a glutton at an all-you-can-eat buffet. Models get thinner and thinner—and younger and younger. Marketers may be trying to appeal to the baby boomers, but much of that appeal is geared toward telling them how to preserve their youth.

Youth—larger-than-life billboards scream it; glossy, perfumed, full-page ads bark it; TV reinforces it; radio shouts it; teen, beauty, health, and fashion magazines glamorize it; and the high-profile fashion world worships it.

Youth—wrinkle-free, sun-kissed, cellulite-absent, white-toothed, snug-fitting youth. Forget that the baby boomers might have money, power, privilege, and wisdom—youth is getting all the press. As a result, the average woman in the United States is seriously concerned about her skin and how it looks—to the point of seeking professional help to do something about it.

Part of that is vanity, and part of it is longevity. Both are valid reasons. As a result, the cosmetic skin-care business has become a multibillion dollar industry, with anti-aging treatments becoming the star products on the professional beauty horizon.

Sales of high performance, anti-aging skin-care products are growing strongly, at approximately 30 percent a year. Demand is driven by aging baby boomers who want to reduce and/or eliminate wrinkles and by younger people who hope to prevent signs of aging. The latest, most innovative skin-care products are cosmeceuticals (which harness the power of science) and botanicals (which are plant-based); these preparations command premium prices.

The trend is strong and only growing stronger, with new products flooding the market every year. Some of these products are bogus, blatant rip-offs; many are fine, outstanding products; and some are absolutely top-notch. How can you tell the difference among them all without getting a medical degree?

This chapter is all about the fancy lotions and potions that you see in the fashion magazines, sample at the makeup counter, and hear about on television. What works? What doesn't? What's worth the money, and what's simply worth a pass?

We'll not only tell you which products we recommend, we'll also give you the tools to decipher fact and fiction for yourself. Our goal here is not just to give you an insider's tour of the beauty and cosmetics industry but also to leave you with enough information so that you can trust yourself to make wiser choices.

Spending Money in Pursuit of Perfection

It's easy to say that cosmetic surgery and nonsurgical procedures are more popular than ever, but what does that really mean? How does that translate into the way modern women live their lives and, just as important, spend their hard-earned money?

The average middle- to upper-class woman in the United States spends thousands of dollars in a lifetime in pursuit of the "perfection" that is portrayed by the models who are pictured on cosmetic packages and in their marketing support materials. This isn't coincidental. In fact, it is widely known from marketing research that women are more likely to buy a product "from" someone who is attractive rather than from an average-looking woman who probably looks more like the consumer.

As we learned in the first chapter of this book, beauty can sometimes be a curse, but current research shows that attractive people do, in fact, earn more money, become more successful, and find more happiness in romance. It's only natural that we would want to be part of that "in" crowd of happy, rich, successful people.

The effect is subliminal; we apparently believe that the "appearance magic" is in the jar at hand and not in the stars or the genes. When it comes to marketing, the U.S. skin-care industry is the unbridled queen, reigning over a kingdom of adoring subjects who worship her every decree—and scoop up every new product.

SOAP: HOW MUCH IS TOO MUCH?

We often take our basic, day-to-day soap for granted. What brand do you use? Are you loyal to one brand? If so, why? If not, why not? These questions and others should be of some concern to you as we make our way through the care of your face.

Why should you be so concerned? If soaps are too alkaline, as many are these days, they can disrupt the epidermis (the outer layer of the skin) and cause flare-ups. Janice Markley, a top consultant for Noevir skin-care products, explains, "Soap is made from fats and alkali solution. These harsh ingredients can strip oils from the skin, leaving it dry and irritated. Soap can also leave a residue when it reacts with calcium, magnesium, and other minerals sometimes present in water; this film can irritate skin further. Soap has a built-in incompatibility with skin. Soap's pH is generally too alkaline (meaning the pH level is greater than 7). Our skin is slightly acidic, with a pH of 5 to 6. The pH of most bar soaps is around 10. Although your skin might feel clean, this change in the skin's pH can leave you with a tight feeling."

If you're looking for quick answers—and an even quicker recommendation—to help cure your soap-caused ills, Dove is still the gold standard, the brand against which everything is measured in soap studies.

If marketing can be so effective for sales, is there any need for the truth? The answer lies in the marketing value of the truth: if science can prove it, then the marketing folks will make sure that you know about it.

We are the most technologically driven culture in history, and as a result, science sells. In the last decade, skin-care and cosmeceutical companies have pushed for scientific credibility in a way that was previously ignored. Scientific studies (good ones and bad ones) are now commonplace.

Such is the problem with science; with the entire marketing hubbub, it's getting harder and harder to separate the blue-ribbon science from the bluff. In our consumer culture, where information is delivered in bite-size nuggets and on the go, like prepackaged junk food, it's easy to overlook the more salient points of a scientific declaration in favor of the bottom line: results.

For instance, the following claim might sound impressive at first: "A recent study indicates that daily use of Petal Fresh face cream resulted in skin that felt 45 percent younger—and looked twice as radiant!"

Thanks to clever packaging and plenty of spin from the wordsmiths back at the home office, the pseudo-study sounds great. If we look a little deeper and stare a little longer, however, more questions than answers start to surface:

- Who did the study? A respected research team at a recognized university or a nonpartisan government agency? Or was it some "consumer group" secretly funded by the makers of Petal Fresh?
- How many people participated in the study? A thousand? A hundred? Ten?
- Were the subjects the same age as the people who are most likely to buy the product?
- How long did the subjects use the product?
- What were the side effects?
- 45 percent younger than what?
- "Felt younger" by whom?
- What was the operational definition of "radiant"?
- How much change is actually represented by "twice as" much? Such wording often masks very minimal results. After all, 2 is "twice as much" as 1. It is one of the most common deceptive strategies in statistics. (For example, "Decaffeinated coffee has only half as much caffeine as regular coffee." In reality, that just means 2 percent instead of 4 percent!)

In other words, all studies are not created equal. In this case, the study must be evaluated in light of potential conflicts of interest. Nevertheless, real scientific advances are being made.

Identifying Good and Bad Products

How do you separate fact from hype and know which products actually do something for your face? It is not easy; there is no exact formula for finding out the truth. One thing is for certain, however: the time-honored answer provided by dermatologists—"Just use plain soap, a good sunscreen, and the cheapest creams and lotions, because the pricier product is no better than the one from your local drugstore"—is no longer true.

In fact, advances are being made—and plenty of them. Walk into the research and development lab for any top cosmetics company, and you might think you took a wrong turn and wound up at NASA!

We all know that we should take better care of our skin. The market has responded with a slew of new products to meet that need, for both beautification and protection.

Relying on your grandmother's sunscreen and your grandfather's soap will most likely get you your grandparents' skin. The newer, superior products are expensive, however, due to the cost of laboratory research, clinical trials, patent applications (in a few instances), and widespread marketing.

THE ROLE OF COSMETICS

Cosmetics can help to improve your appearance, but first you must understand what they *cannot* do. There is a common misconception that dryness of the skin causes aging. This leads people to think that moisturizing the skin is essential to prevent aging. Reversing dryness makes the skin look and feel better, but it does nothing to slow the aging process. Moisturizers, regardless of what they contain and how much they cost, will *not* stop or reverse aging.

What Science Means for Your Skin

There are two problems a product must tackle before either of us will recommend it to our patients or, for that matter, to you:

- **Crossing the barrier layer.** Your skin is designed not just to make you look beautiful or show your age; your skin is designed to protect you from myriad external factors that your body doesn't want you to experience: harmful UV rays, weather, dust, pollution, and even harsh and harmful chemicals. Consider your skin to be your body's living force field. It's not easy getting past the barrier layer (the stratum corneum) of human skin, yet that is exactly what any new, scientifically developed and professionally manufactured skin-care product must do if it is to deliver the results it has promised.

- **The vehicle you're using.** No, we're not talking about cars here. When scientists, cosmetologists, or even dermatologists talk about "the vehicle" in skin care, we're referring to the material with which the active ingredient is mixed, which carries it through the epidermis (the outer layer of the skin) and then releases it at just the right times to the appropriate target. Serums, lotions, creams, gels, and capsules are the vehicles that a product can use to get into your system and do what it's designed to do. However, not all vehicles are suitable for all products. Worse still, when a product is tested in a test tube and achieves amazing results, that does not always mean that the results will translate to effective skin care; this is because of the issues of skin-barrier penetration and effective vehicle activity.

Another issue is herbs. When labels talk about "herbs"—using phrases like "all natural," "herbal supplement," "energy from herbs," and so on—this means that considerable manufacturing quality is required to yield an effective product. After all, most herbs contain fifty to sixty different naturally occurring chemicals, so questions like "Which part is of use?" and "How is it manufactured?" and "How is it grown?" are essential to efficacy. For instance, a skin-care ingredient that has been widely used in the past five years is green tea. The polyphenols contained in green tea are very effective antioxidants.

Thus, how do you know if a new product is effective? How can you tell if those glowing testimonials and professionally photographed "before" and "after" photos really illustrate the results that an average consumer might get? The answer is simple: try the split-face comparison.

If you use a product on one side of your face for three months and don't use it on the other side for the same duration, you may see the results in the mirror. Then you'll know what's fact and what's fiction. We know that most people won't undergo this rigorous exercise so in this book we will try to clarify which products actually do have an impact.

A Change Is Going to Come— Maybe

So far, in this chapter, we've talked a lot about skin-care products: the good, the bad, and the ugly. The chances are, however, that you're still confused. That's because there is so much new technology out there, making so many new products, discoveries, and even delivery systems—serums, potions, lotions, capsules, oils—that it's hard to keep up. We can't promise to categorize— or even list—every skin-care product in this chapter, but we can at least simplify the search by classifying these products into the following two categories:

1. **Rejuvenating change.** This category consists of reparative skin-care products, which attack symptoms: fine lines, discoloration, spots, wrinkles, and so on. These lotions and potions are what you want if you're actively looking to change something in particular about your skin.
2. **Postponing aging change.** This category consists of preventive skin-care products, which work on maintaining what you already have: the luster of youth. These products prevent wrinkles from becoming prominent and provide proper support for clean, healthy skin. Some are designed not so much to change your face for the better but simply to prevent changes from happening for the worse.

A Reparative Skin-Care Regimen

The glow of youth is lost over the years as the top layer of the epidermis becomes thick and opaque. Some skin-care products actually do create change. For instance, they can help to restore the luster of the skin on the outside and create better skin health from the inside. They include the following products:

- **NeoStrata.** Hydroxy acids are one example of skin-care products that actually produce a direct, measurable change: younger, glowing skin. The effect of hydroxy acid is twofold: it produces a smoother texture and color, and it helps acne-prone skin. Although there are many hydroxy acid companies, we use NeoStrata, with its glycolic-based products (see the photograph below), as our example because it was founded and managed by Dr. Eugene Van Scott and Dr. Ruey Yu, who are the world's recognized experts in glycolic acid research.

- **RevaléSkin cream.** Brought to market only in 2007, RevaléSkin cream utilizes the benefits of caffeine to, as the company's slogan says, "wake up your skin." RevaléSkin cream, an antioxidant derived from CoffeeBerry (a concentrated form of the red fruit of the coffee plant), reduces

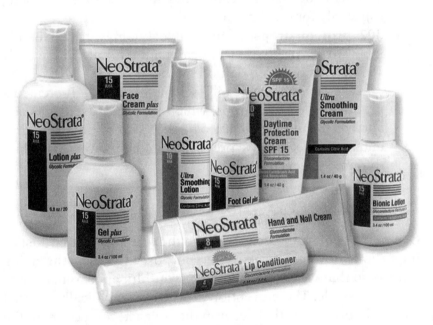

An array of
NeoStrata products

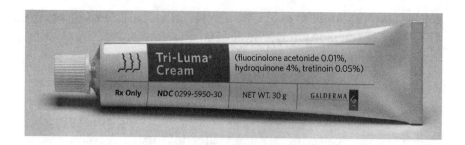

Tri-Luma Cream

lines that are a result of moderate sun damage. RevaléSkin is the first professional line of anti-aging skin care that we are aware of that contains CoffeeBerry. Recent studies have shown that even coffee drinkers—who ingest the bean, not the berry—seem to have a lower instance of internal diseases.

- **Tri-Luma.** Tri-Luma (see the photograph above) is the most widely used prescription bleaching agent in the United States. It contains three prime ingredients: 4 percent hydroquinone, tretinoin, and a topical steroid. This product is excellent for color irregularities in photo-damaged skin, especially for darker skin.

- **302 protein drops**. A topical technology began in the laboratories of pharmaceutical giant Eli Lilly in the early 1990s. This research of more than a decade yielded a spin-off company of former Lilly scientists in 2004. It created a product called 302 Drops, which is derived from avocado and has the unique ability to thicken skin—both the dermis and the epidermis. We prescribe it to help reverse the skin-thinning effects of age.

A Preventive Skin-Care Regimen

One purpose of skin care is to make the skin look better. Just as important, however, is its other purpose: to delay the aging process so that we can maintain our youthful appearance for as long as possible. The prevention of wrinkles is typically focused on the abnormalities that occur in the collagen component of the dermis. Other elements of the dermis include elastic fibers, hyaluronic acids, and blood vessels. These last three are targets of some products as well, yet it is the collagen stimulation factors of cosmeceutical creams and lotions that have received the attention of the skin-care professional and the public.

Retin-A, an acne preparation developed in the late 1960s, was shown to stimulate collagen to such an extent that biopsy studies showed youthful collagen being generously deposited over months. Tretinoin, Retin-A's active ingredient (and also found in Renova), quickly became the gold standard for collagen creams. It held the throne until the early 1990s, when several competitors arrived. Currently, we recommend the following powerful preventive skin-care lines that have been proven by outstanding clinical research:

- **Neova (copper peptide).** Since 1999, copper peptide creams have been considered undoubtedly among the most effective wrinkle prevention creams available. They have been shown in several independent medical school studies to stimulate collagen at almost twice the rate of Retin-A and Renova. Neova offers a wide array of products (see the photograph below).

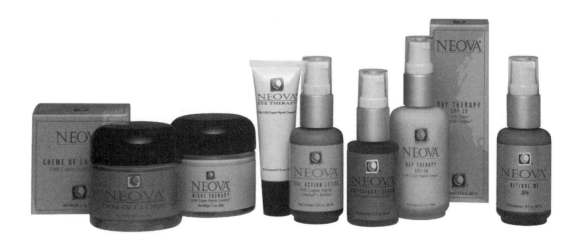

An array of Neova products

- **NIA 24** Niacinamide-based NIA 24 (see the illustration below), which was tested at the National Cancer Institute, may be able to reverse DNA damage. This product is very important for people with fair skin who have had sun damage—even severe damage. We have noticed, with numerous individuals, a softening of color irregularity and a reduction in scaling, precancerous growths. Therefore, this product serves a unique purpose by perhaps reducing the prevalence of skin cancer in people who use it while also reducing another major effect of the sun: wrinkles.
- **Antioxidants.** Cells are attacked by harmful elements called *free radicals*. One of the leading theories on skin aging is that it can be prevented by stopping the formation of free radicals with antioxidants (which are considered "free-radical scavengers"). Antioxidant skin-care products have increasingly assumed center stage. There are numerous antioxidants used in skin-care products, including vitamins

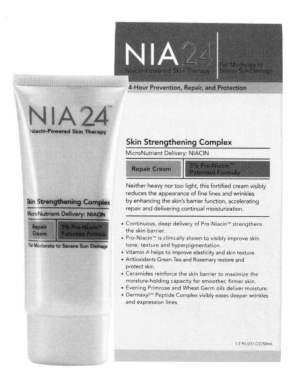

An ad for NIA 24

(C and E) and herbal and green tea extracts (polyphenols). This list is likely to expand rapidly and may even have value in preventing skin cancer. Following are some common antioxidant products:

> **Replenix.** Replenix is our most recommended antioxidant preventive skin-care product. It contains green tea–derived polyphenols, which are known to be strong antioxidants.
>
> **Citrix—Vitamin C.** Vitamin C is the most plentiful antioxidant in human skin and a potent anti-inflammatory agent. Our recommended vitamin C–based antioxidant skin-care system, Citrix, is commonly used on acne-prone and oily skin because it functions as an astringent.
>
> **Persimmon leaf.** The leaf of the persimmon plant contains tannins (which are also found in wine) and has skin-lightening and collagen-stimulating capacities. We are looking at new and recent skin-care developments in this area.

- **Broad-spectrum sunscreens.** Sunscreen application is perhaps the most important preventive measure for sun damage and aging. See the following section for a detailed discussion.

Other Skin Care Products in the News

We have outlined many different skin-care systems in this chapter. You are probably wondering about all the other creams, lotions, and potions that you have used in the past with good results or have seen in national magazines and on television. There are many great skin-care systems on the market, and we have obviously not tried to cover all of them. We have put forth a group that we believe produce results in our clinical practices. We do not have a financial interest in any of these companies. These are cutting-edge as well as time-tested products, with sound scientific research to back them. In this section we will talk about some other products that you may have heard about that are good products but that no longer pass muster, in our clinical opinions:

- **Retin-A and Renova.** The active ingredient here is tretinoin. These were the gold standards for collagen-stimulating (antiwrinkle) cosmeceuticals for many years. Recently manufactured products appear to be superior, however.
- **SkinMedica Growth Factor.** According to a press release from the American Society for Dermatologic Surgery, "Growth factors refer to a variety of natural protein substances that facilitate the communication between damaged and healthy cells and thus increase the rate of new cell growth. It is a proven treatment for chronic, non-healing skin wounds such as extensive burns and ulcerations caused by diabetes." We have concerns, however, about the theoretical possibility of the stimulation of skin cancers by these growth factors.

While the above products have some merit, we believe that our recommended products are superior.

Does Mother Nature Know Best? Organic Beauty Products

Another trend sweeping the nation right now is the green craze, in which the environment meets commerce, and we are being treated to nothing less than a revolution of products that are eco-friendly. From recycled plastics to long-lasting lightbulbs to soy milk, life is getting better—and Earth-friendlier—one product at a time.

The cosmetic industry is no different, and we have seen more new products that are labeled *organic* reach the market than ever before. As active proponents of home health care, we welcome and embrace this growing trend.

Organic lotions and potions feature a variety of natural and

Earth-friendly ingredients, from natural exfoliants like mineral clays, black mud, and apricot kernel meal to gentle natural cleansers such as French green clay and chamomile flower powder. We say the fewer chemicals, the better.

So much of what we promote is prevention, and the all-natural products that work are genuinely concerned with preventing damage from the sun, the wind, and pollution while also creating stronger, fresher, and younger skin by increasing moisture, cleanliness, and immunities.

Although there are far too many new and untested products for us to examine here, let alone recommend, any health-food store or natural-cosmetics counter staff can help you to begin your quest for organic products.

Among the many benefits of organics are that they are never tested on animals, they are friendlier to the environment because they are pesticide- and chemical-free, and they do not add unnatural toxins and chemicals to your body. Whether they work better than nonorganic products depends on the active ingredients, the concentration, and many complexities.

Nevertheless, organic does not guarantee efficacy. Mother Nature is not as benign as one might think. Even natural ingredients, when not combined accurately or when measured poorly, can create strong, almost toxic reactions to the sensitive skin of the face, the ears, and the neck.

As professionals who have seen too many clients get scammed by misleading labels and unsafe trends, we encourage you to proceed with caution. Just as we advise people when they are switching from one product to another, we caution you to apply this simple three-step plan:

1. **Make sure the product is actually organic.** Just as some diet sodas or artificially flavored juices claim to be "all natural" yet are anything but, unscrupulous companies and savvy advertisers have noticed the green trend and have quickly slapped labels that say "all-natural" on products that are not. Read the label closely, shop at health-food stores, read up on the products, do comparisons, and bug the store's help for real information. Look for the U.S.

Department of Agriculture (USDA) organic seal on the product; without it, a product is not *certified* organic, no matter what manufacturer claims appear on the label.

2. **Test the results before switching.** Americans have a tendency to be all or nothing. Before we start a diet, we throw out all the junk food. When we clean out the garage, we're as likely to get rid of family heirlooms as we are broken toasters and dried-up mops. Your face requires different treatment. The latest organic product or homemade remedy from the nearest health-food store or beautician may work better than any synthetic or commercial product you've ever tried—great! We'll be the first to recommend it and use it, if so. If not, you'll be kicking yourself for throwing out all those other expensive lotions and potions before you did a test run first. We recommend trying the product on a small patch of skin, such as the back of your hand or the underside of your arm, for a day or two before trying the product on the sensitive areas of your face or neck.

3. **Is it right for you?** Even if an organic beauty product is effective, it might still not be right for you. Some products are harsh and dry out your skin, and some don't dry it out enough. Others aren't convenient, don't store well, and cost twice as much as the alternative. Trust us, if something is organic *and* effective, it's not going anywhere; the chances are that over time the product will be perfected and , then, at a later date, it could be better for you. Until then, stick with what works and simply stay on top of the research. It never hurts to keep trying different products until you've found the magic recipe for youthful skin and ageless beauty—organic or otherwise.

An Experiment on Ourselves

To aid the cause of scientific discovery, Dr. Hamilton used one of our recommended skin-cream products on the left eye region, where there is a greater degree of sun damage and wrinkling on most people from sun exposure while driving. He used it on the more difficult side in an attempt to have the most obvious, positive results possible.

By applying the product on a daily basis every morning for three months, he hoped to show fewer lines on the cared-for side of the face than on the uncared-for side.

The proper procedure is to apply a sunscreen in the morning after the skin-care regimen and then a skin cream after using it at night. The author admits that because of his tight schedule he cut corners; he applied the skin cream in the morning without using any sunscreen.

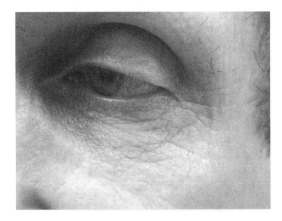

Left eye, with skin-care cream

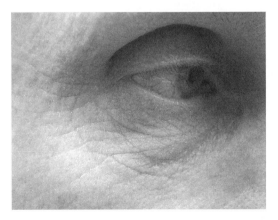

Right eye, without skin-care cream

Sunscreens: What You Don't Know Can Hurt You (and What You Think You Know Can, Too!)

Of all the misconceptions there are about skin-care products, few are of more concern to us than the confusion about sunscreens. What should you know? How much should you know? What does UV really mean, and what's this about UVA?

Ultraviolet (UV) radiation, according to the National Cancer Institute, is "invisible rays that are part of the energy that comes from the sun. UV radiation also comes from sun lamps and tanning beds. UV radiation can damage the skin and cause

SUNSCREEN AND THE VITAMIN D CONTROVERSY

You might not know much about vitamin D, but your body sure does. The many benefits of vitamin D include healthy teeth and bones, a strong immune system, and even reduced blood pressure.

Vitamin D is the one vitamin that our bodies are efficient at making—when our skin is exposed to direct sunlight. For most of us, getting enough vitamin D isn't a problem. Around fifteen minutes of sun exposure several times a week is all that most people need to get enough vitamin D.

Therein lies the rub. Sun can be harmful to your skin, but not getting enough vitamin D can be harmful to your body. Many doctors say that we should avoid the sun at all costs, because it is the best way to avoid harmful UV rays. Other doctors refute this claim; they highly recommend that we get ten to fifteen minutes of sun per day—or at least a few times a week—to ensure that we get enough vitamin D for good health.

There *is* a solution: you can obtain plenty of vitamin D for a strong, healthy body merely by adding certain foods to your current diet: dairy products—cheese, cream, butter, and fortified milk—plus fresh fish and fortified cereals. Getting enough vitamin D could just be the best part of your day!

melanoma and other types of skin cancer."

UV radiation that reaches the Earth's surface is made up of two types of rays, called UVA and UVB rays. UVB rays are more likely than UVA rays to cause sunburn, but UVA rays pass deeper into the skin. Scientists have long thought that UVB radiation can cause melanoma and other types of skin cancer. They now think that UVA radiation may add to skin damage that can lead to skin cancer and cause premature aging. For this reason, skin specialists recommend that people use sunscreens that reflect, absorb, or scatter both kinds of UV radiation.

A sunscreen's sun protection factor, or SPF, number measures the blockage of, or protection from, UVA rays, but these are only part of the potentially damaging rays that come from the sun. Having a high SPF number with minimal UVA protection is like putting six locks on the front door and leaving the back door open.

A sunscreen's sun protection factor, or SPF, number measures the blockage of, or protection from, UVB rays only. Having a high SPF number with minimal UVA protection is like putting six locks on the front door and leaving the back door open.

UVA rays pigment (cause spots) more than UVB rays. Both rays cause damage, and even more so in combination. An additional factor for measuring UVA protection is due soon, after many years of discussion within the FDA.

According to the Environmental Working Group, a nonprofit organization, in 2007, "Our comprehensive scientific review indicates that 84% of 838 sunscreen products offer inadequate protection from the sun, or contain ingredients with significant safety concerns."

UNDERSTANDING NORMAL SKIN

The best way to approach this question is to understand what goes wrong—and where. The outer layer of the skin, the epidermis, is divided into four sublayers, but for our purposes, the epidermis is the thin (about one-tenth of a millimeter) outer layer that people see when they look at your face. It takes part in wrinkling, to some degree, but its biggest contribution to the appearance of aging is its roughness, color irregularity, and loss of luster.

FOUR KEY FACTORS IN AVOIDING
UVB AND UVA DAMAGE

Our skin would look so much better for so much longer if only we could stay out of the sun entirely. However, most of us are out of luck in that regard. The sun is out there, lurking around every corner and waiting for us high overhead, sending down harmful UVB and UVA rays every time we leave the house, get in or out of the car, stop for lunch, or just take a walk around the block.

If we can't (or don't want to) avoid the sun, how can we at least protect ourselves from it? We have instituted a four-part rule that we encourage all our patients to follow:

1. **Wear it.** Clothing can be a huge asset in protecting your skin from the sun. Hats should always be in fashion, particularly if you are a sun lover—and even in addition to your strongest sunscreen. Long-sleeved shirts are also helpful. There are even several clothing lines devoted to the production of garments with a higher than normal SPF rating.

2. **Avoid it.** The best thing you can do, in our opinion, is to avoid the sun as much as possible. If you are searching for a tan, get it from a bottle. Self-tanners that contain dihydroxyacetone as the active ingredient are generally recognized as quite safe. At least one of the authors has been sprayed at a chic tanning salon near his Beverly Hills office.

3. **Time.** UVB and UVA rays are the most harmful when they're at their peak, typically from eleven in the morning until about three in the afternoon. We add an hour to each end of that rule and caution people to stay out of the sun from ten until about four. If you can't (or won't) avoid the sun altogether, you should try to go out when it is least powerful.

4. **Apply it.** Use the skin-care and sunscreen products—relying heavily on zinc-based protection from UVA rays—mentioned in this chapter liberally: every two to four hours and every time you go out into the sun for an extended period. As we tell our patients, "Even the best sunscreen doesn't work if you don't apply it!"

Using these four rules doesn't mean that you're completely protected or off the hook from UVB and UVA damage, but it does mean that you're protecting yourself in four ways that really add up to doing everything possible in your best interest.

What can you do? Whom can you trust? Following is a list of several of the most recent and cutting-edge products that help to protect you from both UVB and UVA rays:

- **Zinc oxide**: To equip yourself with the most protection on the market today, we suggest full-blockage, zinc-containing sunscreen. Until 2007, zinc stood alone as the only true broad-spectrum UVA and UVB protection. Z-Silc is our recommended zinc-based sunscreen.
- **Neutrogena products**: A new product on the market, Neutrogena Ultra Sheer Dry-Touch Sunblock, which comes in SPF 55 and SPF 70, is a dermatologist-tested formula that contains Helioplex technology, the latest breakthrough in UV protection. Helioplex contains avobenzone and oxybenzone. These ingredients effectively block UVA in addition to the traditional UVB rays. Be aware when you go to purchase Neutrogena sunscreens, because they have lines that do not contain Helioplex.
- **LaRoche-Posay:** In early 2007, this company introduced a product similar to Neutrogena's. It contains Mexoryl, which appears to be equally effective in blocking UVA and UVB rays.

A Skin-Care Regimen

In addition to the products we apply and procedures we use in our offices, we suggest a proven system of at-home care to combat the effects of aging on the skin. A skin-care regimen should be individualized, with each person's particular skin type in mind. You and your skin-care medical specialist should work together to come up with what is right for you. In the table on page 84, we have created some examples of a skin-care regimen based on the major skin types.

A typical daily regimen would include reparative as well as preventive skin care systems, applied in the morning and the evening (note that morning and evening applications can be reversed, with the exception of sunscreen, which should be applied in the morning). A gentle cleanser of approximately neutral pH (such as Dove or Neova Herbal Wash) should also be used in the morning and at night before the first application of the products. You should wait fifteen minutes between skin-care product applications. Use this as a guide to discuss this matter with your physician.

SKIN CARE REGIMEN BASED ON SKIN TYPE

Ethnicity/ Skin Type	Preventative[a]		Reparative[a]	
Caucasian (fair to medium pigmentation)	AM:	Replenix serum NIA 24/7; Z-Silc Sunblock[b]	AM:	RevaléSkin
	PM:	Neova Night Therapy; Neova Eye Therapy	PM:	NeoStrata Bionic Lotion (every other night); 302 Drops (for neck and hands)
Caucasian (darker pigmentation)	AM:	Replenix serum NIA 24/7; Z-Silc Sunblock[b]	AM:	NeoStrata 10% Smoothing Crème
	PM:	Beauty rest	PM:	Tri-Luma (4 percent hydroquinone, tretinoin, and steroid) or 4 percent hydroquinone (for brown spots) 302 Drops (for neck and hands)
African American	AM:	Citrix (Vitamin C); Z-Silc Sunblock[b]	AM:	NeoStrata 10% Smoothing Crème
	PM:	Various creams containing arbutin or persimmon leaf extracts	PM:	Tri-Luma (4 percent hydroquinone, tretinoin, and steroid) or 4 to 8 percent hydroquinone (for brown spots)
Hispanic	AM:	Citrix (Vitamin C); Z-Silc Sunblock[b]	AM:	RevaléSkin (Tues., Thurs., Sat., Sun.); NeoStrata 10% Smoothing Crème
	PM:	Neova Night Therapy	PM:	Tri- Luma (4 percent hydroquinone, tretinoin, and steroid) or 4 percent hydroquinone (for brown spots)
Asian	AM:	Citrix (vitamin C); Z-Silc Sunblock[b]	AM:	NeoStrata 10 percent Smoothing Crème
	PM:	Beauty rest	PM:	Tri-Luma (4 percent hydroquinone, tretinoin, and steroid) or 4 percent hydroquinone (for brown spots)

[a] Wash with a cleanser of approximately neutral pH (Dove or Neova Herbal Wash) morning and night before first application of products; wait fifteen minutes between skin-care product applications.
[b] May substitute Neutrogena (with Helioplex) or La Roche-Posay (with Mexoryl).

Adjunctive Measures for Better Skin

Finally, we should note that we have entered the era of hormonal manipulation in healthy individuals for the sole purpose of intervening in the normal aging process. The classic example is systemic human growth hormone (HGH), along with testosterone supplementation in males. These hormones may have a beneficial effect on skin elasticity and lean body mass, but there are concerns about the possible stimulation of internal cancers.

We do not recommend the use of HGH, because research information is still lacking. The claim for its beneficial effects relies on only one study, done in 1990 by Dr. Daniel Rudman and others, in which twenty-one men were treated for six months without any long-term follow-up. Dr. Rudman, before his death in 1993, warned that the doses he used were too high to be considered safe and that more studies are necessary before HGH can be recommended for widespread use.

An approach to systematic aging that appears safer and that presently has more evidence for efficacy is the oral administration of antioxidant vitamins and other supplements such as vitamins C and E, alpha lipoic acid, coenzyme Q10, and L-arginine. We encourage our readers to seek out scientific information on dosages.

FREE RADICALS

Free radicals are molecules gone bad through their coupling with oxygen. Evidence suggests that this process induces most of the cellular changes associated with aging.

5

The Big Three

Wrinkles, Spots, and Roughness

Have you ever looked in the mirror and wondered where those brown spots came from? Have you ever wondered when, why, and how your skin got so rough all of a sudden? Furthermore, what's up with those fine lines?

In this chapter we get straight to "the big three," as we—and most people—see them: wrinkles (fine lines), (brown and red) spots, and rough skin. On the following pages, we introduce the most popular and effective treatments for them; these procedures are well known in the industry.

Our in-depth analysis of today's top products gives you a veritable "consumer's report" of the latest advances in dermatological and cosmetic procedures, including the following:

- Lasers
- Chemical peels
- Intense pulsed light (IPL)
- Depigmenting mask
- Microdermabrasion

Wrinkles (Fine Lines)

Traditionally, there have been two general ways to treat wrinkles: deep chemical peels (for centuries) and lasers (for about a dozen years). We will reverse the chronology in the following discussion, since laser technology developments are moving more rapidly than peels and are supplanting, to some degree, the use of peels for wrinkles. Although superficial (glycolic and others) and medium-depth peels are still widely used to help with glow and roughness, they do not penetrate deeply enough to help with wrinkles.

Lasers

People often speak of wanting (or not wanting) "the laser" for this problem or that. In fact, there is no one laser; there are dozens of laser categories or types, and for each of these types, there are dozens of brands (companies), so there are hundreds of names to track. This can be clearly understood, however, if we work back from those hundreds of names and just understand what problems they treat and the laser type (category) that is applied for the treatment.

The easiest route for understanding lasers is to see it from what you, as the patient, need. In the following section we will therefore highlight your problem and then talk about the two hundred laser answers.

In the 1990s, a revolution was started by the advent of a new type of technology. The CO_2 laser, which is now manufactured by more than ten companies, was modified to allow treatment of (only) facial wrinkles. Its results were striking; the skin was literally transformed by this *ablative* (which means "burning") technology. Further modifications in ablative approaches were instituted with erbium lasers (once again, there are several companies, with catchy names, that make them).

Erbium was sometimes referred to as a "cool" laser, even though it was cool only by comparison to the very hot CO_2 lasers. The erbium lasers avoided the major side effects of the CO_2 lasers, such as loss of color (usually permanent) in a small percentage of cases. However, the CO_2 laser had the advantage of tightening the skin, particularly around the eyes, which the erbium lasers could not do.

Although a large number of people opted for these two types of laser procedures in the mid-1990s with excellent results, there was a decrease in the frequency of usage around 2000 due to the prolonged downtime associated with their use. Full-face procedures required the patient to be treated under conscious sedation (twilight anesthesia), wear bandages, and follow wound-care instructions. The downtime before being able to return to work was about ten days. Thus, a search for no or little downtime began. The hope was to bypass injury to the epidermis and merely stimulate collagen production in the dermis by selective injury. Soon, several *nonablative* lasers, such as the NLite and the CoolTouch, appeared. These lasers had no downtime, but they gave slow results, thus requiring numerous repeat treatments.

These lasers are still frequently used, and there has even been something of a resurgence in the application of the CO_2 laser. We find the latter to be of special value in improving wrinkles of the lower eyelids while also tightening the loose skin of the lower lids, which is otherwise very difficult to manage with either lasers or surgery.

An answer to the need for "no downtime" in resurfacing (wrinkle removal) arrived in the end of 2004 with the release of the SR750 Fraxel laser by Reliant Technologies. This laser, developed by R. Rox Anderson, a professor of dermatology at Harvard Medical School's Wellman Center for Photomedicine, was revolutionary in its approach.

By dividing each laser beam discharge into thousands of nanobeams, microscopic thermal zones were treated on the skin surface with even deeper penetration than that afforded by the CO_2 or erbium lasers. About 20 percent of the surface was hit with each treatment session. It was noted that the distance between the hits was so small that the untreated areas were undetectable. Healing began from the surface, with the epidermal cells regenerating to heal the surface almost immediately.

This enabled two factors:

* The level of penetration could be deeper with Fraxel than with CO_2.
* Areas other than the face could be treated, since healing did not require help from hair follicle cells, which was necessary with CO_2.

Fraxel had additional rejuvenation benefits beyond those of facial wrinkle removal: removal of roughness, improvement of texture, and a smoothing out of color irregularities, including chloasma. With the Fraxel laser, unlike with the CO_2, there have been no reported cases of color loss. Five treatments, spaced two to four weeks apart, are generally recommended (100 percent benefit is achieved with five sessions, although fewer treatments provide some benefit). There is generally no downtime, but some pinkness and dryness may be present for a few days.

A new addition to Fraxel, the SR1500, was approved by the FDA in January 2007 and allows deeper penetration because of higher energy levels. In this new treatment, blue dye is avoided altogether. A third Fraxel device offers fractionated CO_2 technology.

Be aware of the following facts when considering these treatments:

1. Neither the medical literature nor, indeed, the company has offered much proof that the SR1500 yields greater efficacy than the SR750 since no side-by-side studies have been done.
2. The development of fractionated CO_2 devices is a step back in time. The ablative CO_2 lasers of the mid-1990s are certainly more effective for wrinkles than the fractionated lasers are, but the ablative CO_2 lasers require longer downtime as well. The fractionated CO_2 devices, in turn, produce better results than the nonablative fraxelated lasers do, but the latter require virtually no downtime at lower energy levels, whereas the former normally require a three- to five-day healing period.

Other companies have since "fraxelated" their lasers (much like pixels in a digital camera). We believe that they produce results comparable to that of Reliant's Fraxel laser. In addition, there is a movement by some companies to add a CO_2 component to this technology. Lasers that are competitive with the Reliant product include Palomar's Lux 1540/2940, Lumenis's ActiveFX, Affirm's CO2, and Cutera's Pearl.

Ultimately, the choice of laser treatments for wrinkles comes down to weighing the following: how long you are willing to wait for the results, how much downtime you can tolerate, and what you can pay, at least up front.

Fractionated Skin Resurfacing

As we just mentioned, companies other than Reliant (the manufacturer of Fraxel) have made fractionated versions of their lasers. Fractional lasers have advanced the field of skin resurfacing by producing excellent results with minimal downtime.

Fractional lasers deliver columns of light that penetrate down to the dermis without causing damage to the surrounding tissues. The beams actually penetrate deeper than the CO_2 or erbium lasers. The injury within the columns of tissue stimulates the formation of new collagen.

Fractional lasers stimulate quick healing within the surrounding deep tissue, resulting in deep corrections and long-term dermal remodeling. Nonablative fractional lasers such as Lux 1540 require multiple treatments to obtain the desired results. Fractionated CO_2 lasers typically require only one treatment.

What Can Laser Surgery Do for You?

In our practices we are always asked about lasers. Can lasers be used to perform face-lifts, eyelid lifts, brow lifts, or skin resurfacing? What can laser surgery do for you? The answer to the last question depends on the problem at hand and your doctor. Lasers and light-based devices can be successfully used for a variety of skin-related problems that are noted in this chapter, especially fine lines and wrinkles.

The key to your outcome depends on the extent of your aging wrinkles and the person who is holding the laser and how experienced he or she is—or isn't. Facial plastic surgeons and experienced dermatologists are trained in the use of lasers and understand when and how to use them. The surgeon will decide if he or she wants to use a laser and which one would be the best choice for the situation. A fancy laser in inexperienced hands or for the wrong aging problem will not yield good results.

Be aware that there are hundreds of types of lasers (and these fall into about twenty different major categories), each with a different function. Do not consider all lasers equal or let your physician speak in simplified terms, as if all lasers are created equal; do your homework and discuss with your doctor which of these

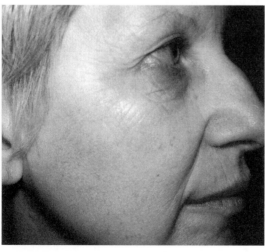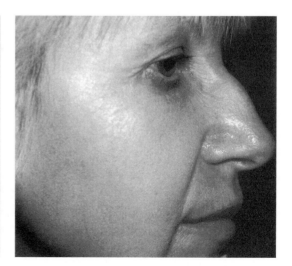

Before and after CO_2, two weeks

hundreds of types of lasers is right for you and your current concerns about aging and skin care.

There are many benefits to cosmetic skin resurfacing. Lasers are able to change tissue without making an incision. Because of laser technology, for instance, major surgery does not have to be performed to treat birthmarks or damaged blood vessels, remove port-wine stains, or shrink facial spider veins. The photos on page 93 show the results of CO_2 laser on one of Dr. Hamilton's patients.

Chemical Peels

The standard chemical peel is a treatment that uses a chemical solution to improve and smooth the texture of the facial skin by removing its damaged outer layers. It is helpful for individuals with facial blemishes, wrinkles, and uneven skin pigmentation. The precise formula that is used can be adjusted to meet each patient's needs.

Chemical peels can also remove precancerous skin growths, soften acne facial scars, and even control acne. It is not a treatment that closes up enlarged pores. Types of chemical peels include the following:

- *Alpha hydroxy acids (AHAs)*, such as glycolic and lactic acids, are fruit acids that are the mildest of the peel formulas and produce light peels. These superficial peels can provide smoother, brighter-looking skin for people who can't spare the time to recover from deeper phenol or trichloroacetic acid (TCA) peels. AHA peels may be used on areas of dryness, uneven pigmentation, and acne. Various concentrations of an AHA may be applied weekly or at longer intervals to obtain the best result. An alpha hydroxy acid, such as glycolic acid, can also be mixed with a facial wash or a cream in lesser concentrations as part of a daily skin-care regimen to improve the skin's texture.
- *Trichloroacetic acid (TCA)* can be used in many concentrations, but it is most commonly used for medium-depth peeling (25 to 30 percent concentration). Fine wrinkles, superficial blemishes, and pigment problems are commonly treated with TCA. The results of TCA peels are more evident than AHA peels but less dramatic and not as long lasting as those of phenol peels. In fact, more than one TCA peel may be needed to achieve the desired result. The recovery from a 30% TCA peel is five to seven days.
- *Phenol* is the strongest of the chemical solutions and produces a deep peel. It is used mainly to treat people with deep facial wrinkles, areas of blotchy or damaged skin caused by sun exposure, or precancerous growths. Since phenol often lightens the treated areas, your skin pigmentation will be a determining factor for whether this is an appropriate treatment for you. Phenol is used primarily on the face; scarring can result if it's applied to the neck or other body areas. Phenol can be a good treatment for leathery and extensively sun-damaged skin in older individuals if it is performed by an experienced physician and if the patient is willing to accept the likelihood of some

lightening of the facial skin, a healing time of seven to ten days, and a relatively high cost.

Although chemical peels are generally considered safe, the word *chemical* should alert you to the fact that there is some risk involved. All facial rejuvenation procedures should be performed by a qualified, experienced dermatologist or plastic surgeon, but this is particularly true for chemical peels. The risks involved with chemical peels range from mild discoloration and discomfort to scarring and infection.

As we age, the accumulated effects of sun exposure, pollutants, acne, and scarring can damage our skin and cause us to look older than we actually are. Such skin damage can be treated with a chemical peel to promote cell growth and produce smoother, clearer skin. However, lasers, because of their more predicable results, are now frequently used in cases where peels were used in the past.

Spots

Brown spots and chloasma (known as the "mask of pregnancy" when it occurs in pregnant women) can be removed effectively by intense pulsed light (IPL) laser-derived treatments, with generally no downtime. The pigment gradually fades but can recur if a full-spectrum sunscreen is not used. In addition, if you are darker Caucasian, Asian, Hispanic, or African-American, your risk of further darkening is slightly higher, although this effect usually fades over the months. A chemical mask, peel, or bleaching cream may be a better approach, at times. *Photo rejuvenation* and *photo facial* are names used to describe IPL. A series of two to five treatments is normally required. A Q-switched Nd:YAG laser can also be used in stubborn cases.

Intense Pulsed Light: Photo Rejuvenation

Intense pulsed light, or IPL, is a popular skin treatment offered by many dermatologists and plastic surgeons wherein a broad

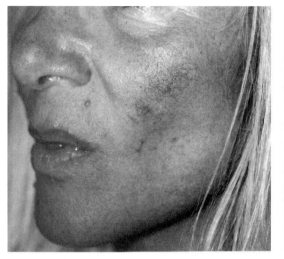
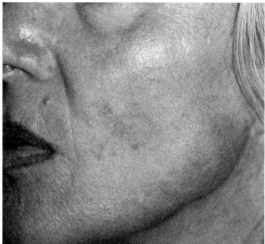

Before IPL   After IPL

spectrum of light is applied to the skin. IPL is used to reverse signs of aging that are caused by exposure to the sun; it can also improve irregular or uneven skin tone, including red and brown spots.

IPL allows your physician to tailor his or her efforts to your unique skin type or irregularity, and the procedure is generally considered to be safe and effective, in the proper hands. If you have a severe problem, the results can be effective and dramatic.

Before the procedure, your physician will apply a topical gel to the area of the skin to be treated and offer you dark glasses as protection from the light given off by the IPL. As the handheld IPL device is applied to your face around the area to be treated, short pulses of light deliver the correct amount of exposure to improve your skin.

Each treatment typically takes between twenty and thirty minutes, and most physicians recommend getting at least five to six treatments, for long-lasting satisfactory results. Generally, the treatments are scheduled once a month for the duration of your choice.

The upside to IPL is that since the treatments are short, safe, and monthly, the downtime is virtually nil. Most people return to work or their routine activities on the day of treatment, and since a treatment doesn't take long, you can schedule appointments even when you don't have a great deal of spare time.

If you have any of the following conditions, you might want to consider IPL treatment:

- Symptoms of rosacea
- Broken veins and capillaries
- Imperfections from sun damage and photo aging

The Caracas Mask

Cosmelan is an excellent pigment-removing alternative to IPL and lasers in certain dark skin types (Latin Americans, Asians, and Iranians), for whom laser technology can actually make

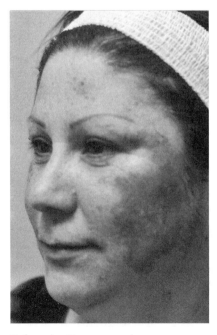

Before the Caracas mask

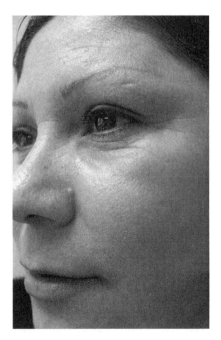

After the Caracas mask

things worse by darkening the very spots that the individuals are attempting to lighten. Cosmelan is a system that uses a chemical mask designed especially for these skin types. This process allows us to remove facial and body brown spots in just a few days.

For more than twenty years, a Caracas plastic surgeon, Dr. Eduardo Grulig, has been effectively treating Latino individuals for melasma and chloasma and other pigment irregularities. A mud mask is applied in the office, and you go home with it on, removing it with water eight hours later.

A very superficial peel occurs for one to two days; you are slightly pink afterward, but this can be easily covered with makeup. Normally, there is no time lost from work. The results

Cosmelan is a truly revolutionary system that uses a chemical mask designed especially for certain dark skin types. This process allows us to remove facial and body brown spots in just a few days.

FOUR TYPES OF AGING, FOUR TYPES OF TREATMENT

As the face ages, there are four different changes that can occur:

Type 1: Wrinkles (fine lines)
Type 2: Furrows (deep expression lines)
Type 3: Laxity (looseness)
Type 4: Atrophy (loss of skin, fat, and bone tissue)

Treatments for type 1 are discussed in this chapter. Treatments for type 2 will be covered in chapter 6, for type 3 in chapters 7 and 8, and for type 4 in chapters 7 and 8. Briefly, the treatments appropriate for each type of aging are as follows:

Type 1: Lasers or deep chemical peels
Type 2: Botox and/or fillers
Type 3: Face-lift for moderate to advanced: Thermage, Titan, ReFirme, and Accent for mild laxity
Type 4: Fillers, multilevel fat grafting, and surgical implants

are virtually immediate, with 75 to 80 percent improvement within a week. The risks are minimal, and a posttreatment bleaching regimen can prevent recurrences and improve results. The only caveat is a possible recent change in the formulation by the company that could have an influence on its effectiveness. The photos on page 98 show an actual patient of Dr. Hamilton's, before and after.

Rough Skin

Microdermabrasion—the process of removing the face's outer layer of dead or damaged skin—is an excellent solution for blemished, wrinkled, rough, or otherwise aged skin.

The procedure involves the mechanical removal of the epidermis by air-driven aluminum oxide crystals. Because the epidermis contains no blood vessels, there is generally no bleeding during microdermabrasion. Treatments must be repeated monthly to maintain the benefits.

6

Injectables and How Long They Last

Let's face it: we live in a fast-paced, drive-through, fast-food, 24/7 world. Newspapers are losing readers because nobody wants to wait until the morning to get yesterday's news. Even nightly news has gone down in the ratings because people want their news all day, every day. As much as we want our questions answered immediately, we want results even sooner than that!

By constantly writing for, appearing in, subscribing to, and devouring the latest medical journals in our fields of specialty, we know what has been approved, what works, what doesn't work, what hasn't been approved, and why. We know that people are always on the hunt for the next procedure, the next product, or the next available appointment to discuss how to prevent or reverse aging. We want to know how a treatment works and how a product has been tested, speak to the researchers who have published the results, and witness firsthand how effective such treatments and products can be. Both of us are often asked by prospective companies to perform initial clinical studies on cutting-edge aesthetic products.

On the other hand, safety, quality, and results are more important than speed. There is far too much risk involved for us to use or recommend a product that has questionable results or adverse side effects that might leave our patients worse off than they were before.

Doctors often get caught up in purchasing devices that have been sold to them with strong marketing but with weak science in order not to miss the patient rush that results from the device company's media advertising. The media, after all, are in the "buzz" business; they do not have the expertise, nor do they usually take the time, to evaluate the technology.

How about your dermatologist? What about your plastic surgeon? If he or she is always hawking the "latest and greatest" treatments, ask about conflict of interest with the particular treatment, inquire about the products' safety ratings and side effects, and even request to read the pertinent literature. Even then, some medical journals could potentially have a conflict of interest because of pharmaceutical support. Most of the top-notch medical journals are peer-reviewed and have excellent ethical standards. In short, make sure you have a trustworthy physician and confidant.

A qualified and trusted physician will always make the answers, results, and even the literature available; our offices are half waiting room, half library. We can't stress enough the value of a good relationship with your physician. It is your job to research, interview, inquire, and experiment until you find a doctor you can trust. That is more important than trying to figure out from your favorite publication which "latest and greatest" device will keep you young again forever. If you pick the right doctor, he or she will pick the right technology for you. Remember, even with major advances, there is no one answer for everyone. Evaluation is the key.

Anyone can offer instant, immediate, or overnight results—just look online or in the classifieds or health section of your local paper for the biggest, boldest advertisements. Before you commit to any new procedure, no matter what its duration, ask yourself—and your physician—the following questions:

- Is the product safe?
- What is the recovery time?
- How long does the treatment take?
- How long does it last?
- Will it still be effective six to twelve months from now—or even two years from now?
- How many people have been treated by you, or elsewhere, with this product, and may I talk to a few?
- Ask your doctor if she or he is receiving any financial perks from the company for using its products.

All new procedures take time to reach the commercial market. Any physician worth his or her salt stays abreast of this information through conferences, journals, seminars, and even continued classwork after hours. Many of the fastest procedures are also the least impressive when it comes to results. By asking these questions and pinning your physician down on the answers, you can be well prepared for any new product or procedure—or even those that have been around for years.

You should be aware of a dynamic that often comes into play with the appearance of a new technology. The Food and Drug Administration (FDA) often approves a device for use with just enough data to prove its efficacy and safety; however, the product's effectiveness and the avoidance of side effects is markedly improved after its release by frequent use in the marketplace (that is, physicians' offices). A good basic rule is to wait a year after the product's release before jumping on the bandwagon. Let the doctors work out the bugs on somebody else.

Trust us, your face is nothing to play around with. Quick,

THE DURATION OF INJECTABLE PRODUCTS

This handy chart will help you to determine how long a particular injectable lasts.

Short-Term (3 to 12 months):
- BOTOX Cosmetic (3 months)
- Collagen products
  - Bovine collagen: Zyderm, Zyplast (3 months)
  - Human-based collagen: Cosmoderm, Cosmoplast (3 months)
  - Porcine collagen: Evolence, Evolence Breeze (6 to 12 months)
- Juvéderm (6 to 12 months)
- Restylane (6 to12 months)
- Perlane (6 to 12 months)
- Fascian (extremely variable; increasing duration with repeat treatments)

Long-Term (more than 12 months):
- Radiesse (1 to 2 years)
- Sculptra (2 to 3 years)
- ArteFill (permanent)
- Silikon 1000 (permanent)

cheap, or shoddy work done on the face has ramifications—both physical and mental—that last long after the botched procedure wears off. As the saying goes, you get only one chance to make a first impression—and it always starts with your face.

In general, we can classify such treatments as either shorter (three to twelve months) or longer (twelve months and longer). Which is which? In this chapter we take a look at two ways to approach facial procedures:

1. **Short and sweet—or short-term (three to twelve months).** Many of the treatments we offer fall into the "short and sweet" category, which means that they last for about three to twelve months and require minimal upkeep to maintain their effectiveness.

2. **A (slightly) longer story—or long-term (more than twelve months).** Other procedures last longer and don't require quite so many office visits to maintain.

There are a few reasons that there are two options. It might be a matter of cost (the shorter the duration, the lower the cost) or that certain fillers are not appropriate for certain areas of the face. In addition, certain aging issues can be addressed only by certain technologies, which have a specific duration of effect (for example, loose skin treated by ThermaCool). Another factor that influences choice is downtime (for example, CO_2 laser resurfacing versus fractionated laser resurfacing).

Short and Sweet: Three to Twelve Months

In this section we discuss the facial treatments that we refer to as "short and sweet": you have to come into the office only every three to twelve months to maintain the effects of these mostly temporary, but quite effective, treatments.

These short-term (three- to twelve-month duration) treatments include the following:

- Botox
- Collagen
- Hyaluronic acids (Restylane, Perlane, Juvéderm)
- Fascian

Although you might recognize some of the products or treatments we discuss here, read carefully, because new advances are often on the horizon, and we like to tell you the scoop behind the scoop, if you know what we mean.

Botox

BOTOX Cosmetic is a purified version of a natural protein, *Clostridium botulinum*, that is derived from bacteria. Administered in very small doses, Botox can relax and smooth deep furrows and lines in the face. There's no recovery time, so you can get back to work or participate in other activities immediately.

BOTOX Cosmetic works by reducing muscle contractions and elevations in the treated area, causing even deep lines and forehead furrows to become smoother and less prominent. There usually is some reduction in the ability to raise the brows or squint. Similar deep expression lines in the middle part of the face (such as "smile lines") *cannot* be treated with Botox, since an inability to move the mouth would result. An exception is the furrows of the lip known as "smoker's lines."

A freeze on expression is sought by many people in order to reduce the progression of the lines that would be created by the expression; however, our actor patients sometimes request to have the ability to emote remain. Such a fine line of therapy may be hard to achieve.

Botox is one of the most popular nonsurgical treatments being performed today, but it is important to have it done by an experienced dermatologist or facial plastic surgeon and not just anyone.

How BOTOX Cosmetic Is Administered

BOTOX Cosmetic is administered as a series of small subcutaneous and intramuscular injections in the desired area. In most cases, no anesthetic is required, although the area may be numbed with an ice pack or a topical anesthetic if you are particularly sensitive.

The procedure itself takes only a matter of minutes, after which you will be able to continue your normal activities. In some cases, you may feel a slight tingling or soreness in the area for a short time, but there should be no serious pain or other side effects. Massage of any temporary swelling is probably not a good idea, for this could potentially disperse the toxins and produce negative side effects.

The effects of Botox begin in about forty-eight hours and can be expected to last up to three months; treatment can be repeated as often as necessary as the effects wear off. Allergan, the maker of BOTOX Cosmetic, estimates that between 4 and 14 percent of individuals are somewhat nonresponsive to Botox.

So-called Botox parties have been highlighted in the media. We think that they're a bad idea; any party that is centered around a toxin stronger than alcohol should be avoided! Although Botox is quite safe, the risk of mistakes increases with the gaiety.

A common cause of confusion among people is the dilution factor. Many are concerned that their doctor is diluting the Botox. In reality, since Botox comes to the physician as a powder, all Botox is diluted. The question is how much. It has been shown that dilution ratios of more than 10 to 1 will reduce the duration of the effects. Any lesser dilutions are chosen by physicians on the basis of how they believe they are personally best able to administer the procedure. You should ask your physician about the number of "units" being utilized. This will allow you to better understand the cost structure and strength of the product.

Botox treatments have been incredibly popular in the last ten years. It is said that there are two Botox treatments performed worldwide for every filler injection with products such as collagen and Restylane. The great irony is the following: treatment of the midface with fillers is actually more important for the aesthetics of aging than the forehead is; the latter is not the focus of another's gaze and can even be covered by bangs. We predict that the emphasis will shift away from botulinum toxin toward the use of fillers. In addition, Reloxin, a new form of botulinum toxin, is expected to be available in 2009.

On the other hand, many new uses for Botox in places other than the forehead have risen in the past few years. These include the reduction of furrows around the lips and on the chin; the temporary correction of downward-turning corners of the mouth ("sad clown" look); and the treatment of neck bands. We also utilize Botox for patients with facial paralysis and to narrow the width of the jaw region in Asian patients who have "masseter hypertrophy."

These uses require caution and expertise, since the functioning of the mouth can be disturbed or there can be difficulty swallowing or holding the head erect as a result. A commonly performed "specialty"/off-label procedure with Botox is a chemical brow lift, which is produced by injecting Botox on the outer portion of the brows, denervating the muscles that lower the brows.

Botox is most commonly used to treat the following conditions:

- **Furrows.** When we use our muscles to form facial expressions—particularly when we smile, squint, frown, or scowl—we contribute to the dynamic wrinkles that form around our lips, on our eyelids, at the corners of our eyes, and between our eyebrows. Since we must all laugh, cry, squint, and otherwise express ourselves throughout the day, there is little we can do to avoid these dynamic wrinkles as we age. They may present themselves as minor features during our youth, but they usually grow more severe with age, eventually becoming more dramatic, until they are considered "furrows." The use of Botox can significantly reduce these dynamic wrinkles, or furrows.

- **Brows.** Your brow is extremely vulnerable to the signs of aging, and, in its broad expanse as we age, it becomes a canvas for the various wrinkles and rough skin that accumulate with time. Your brow can also contribute to the effect of drooping by literally weighing on your upper eye lids. Botox has proven to be highly successful in

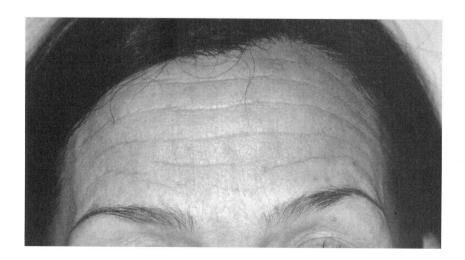

Before Botox
forehead

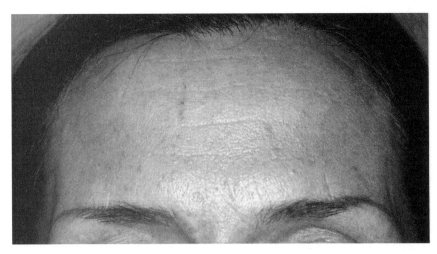

After Botox forehead

improving furrows of the forehead and attending to sagging brows. Brows can also be sufficiently elevated noninvasively by Thermage, if the droop is moderate; if the laxity is advanced, then surgical intervention makes more sense.

Are There Side Effects with Botox?

BOTOX Cosmetic is extremely safe in the hands of an experienced practitioner. Individuals who are pregnant, who are breastfeeding, or who have an active infection should be counseled against its use, however.

The most common side effects include bruising, brow drooping, and lid droop of the treated areas. If the product diffuses to the upper eyelid muscles, the eyelid can droop, resulting in *ptosis*. Other less common side effects include fatigue and facial weakness. Overall, the complication rate is well below 1 percent, and most issues resolve within a few weeks, as the product wears off.

Collagen

Bovine (cow) collagen (Zyderm and Zyplast) first became available in 1981, and for more than twenty years virtually stood alone as the only filler substance used in the United States. It truly initiated noninvasive facial rejuvenation, and its short duration of three months was easily tolerated when no competition was available. Bovine collagen treatment requires skin testing (unlike most fillers that have followed), so immediate gratification on the day of your consultation is not possible if you have not had collagen before. Human-derived collagen (Cosmoderm and Cosmoplast), however, does not require skin testing. It also has a duration of three months. It is grown from human skin under sterile conditions.

The most recent FDA-approved collagen-based product is Evolence. Evolence and (soon to be marketed) Evolence Breeze are Johnson & Johnson products that are composed of porcine (pig) collagen. These products do not require pretesting. They utilize something called GLYMATRIX Technology, which makes it last longer (six months or more) than human-derived and bovine-based collagen. Evolence Breeze, which will most likely be approved by the time this book is published, will have an important role in lip augmentation.

Typical areas of use for collagen include the following:

- Smoothing and filling in wrinkles
- Evening and smoothing pitting, scarring, and other depressions in the skin
- Augmenting and creating fullness in areas such as the lips

Collagen is considered the gold standard for FDA clinical trials for all new fillers. As a result, collagen is the filler against which all new fillers are compared.

How Does Collagen Work?

Collagen is a fibrous protein that is naturally found in your own bones, skin, and cartilage. As we age, the collagen levels in our skin begin to decrease, leading to loss of elasticity and fullness, particularly in the face. Collagen injections will fill in wrinkles, folds and hollows. It is usually injected close to the surface of the skin, and the results will depend on where it is actually injected. Historically, collagen was most commonly used in the treatment of "laugh lines."

How Many Times Must I Be Treated?

Treatment with bovine collagen (Zyplast or Zyderm) requires a test to determine if you are allergic (3 to 5 percent of people are). A wait of one month is required; many physicians perform a second test and wait two weeks, since very rarely is the first test falsely negative. Newer collagen products (Cosmoplast, Cosmoderm, and the Evolence family) do not require allergy testing. The number of individual collagen injections will vary depending on what is being treated. Most individuals will have to repeat injections every three months with bovine and human-derived collagen. Evolence will need to be re-injected every six to twelve months.

Are There Side Effects with Collagen?

Collagen is an extremely safe product with an excellent track record when it's used on the midface, "laugh lines," and lips. Like all fillers, collagen can have some adverse effects, such as bruising, irregularity, overcorrection, undercorrection, and the formation of nodules. However, compared to hyaluronic acids, which will be discussed in the next section, collagen products cause less immediate swelling. Injection is not recommended for the areas under or around the eyes.

How Long Will Collagen Last?

Injectable collagen treatments will fill in depressions or lines and augment soft-tissue features to give you a fresh, glowing, youthful look. Bovine and human-derived collagen are the shortest-lasting fillers, with a duration of three months. Evolence has been reported to last six months or longer.

Hyaluronic Acids

Hyaluronic acids are produced in the body and help to maintain not only skin growth but also volume. As the skin ages and is exposed to environmental pollutants and the sun, the cells lose the ability to produce hyaluronic acid. As a result, the skin begins to lose volume, which often results in the formation of facial wrinkles. Dermal fillers are used by physicians to help temporarily replace lost hyaluronic acid and to restore skin volume.

How Do Hyaluronic Acids Work?

Currently, these acids are approved for use as dermal fillers, and much like the type produced in your own body, these hyaluronic acids help to produce volume and fullness in the aging face. When such acids are injected into skin that is wrinkled or has lost its laxity, they work to create a sense of fullness and volume in the skin; they don't exactly eliminate the furrows, but they do reduce their prominence in the newly full skin.

Hyaluronic acids are used primarily to treat the following:

- "Laugh lines"
- "Marionette lines"
- Cheek and chin volume loss
- The brows
- The glabella (the space between the eyebrows and above the nose)
- Thin lips
- Lower eyelid hollows

How Many Times Must I Be Treated?

Each product that utilizes hyaluronic acid is different; see the various product descriptions below for specific treatment options.

Are There Side Effects with Hyaluronic Acids?

Like collagen products, hyaluronic acids are extremely safe. The most common issues that are encountered with these products include bruising, overcorrection, undercorrection, asymmetry, and nodule formation. If the product is injected superficially under the thin eyelid skin, a bluish hue (known as the *Tyndall effect*) may be visible. Special care must be taken with use under the eyes (that is, in a nonsurgical blepharoplasty). Make sure that your physician has significant expertise in using hyaluronic acid in the eye region.

Unlike other fillers, hyaluronic acids do have a specific antidote if the desired results have not been obtained. *Hyaluronidase* is a product that can break down hyaluronic acids in a safe and expeditious manner.

How Long Will Hyaluronic Acids Last?

The effects will last from six to twelve months, depending on the area of injection.

Restylane and Perlane

Restylane and Perlane are injectable fillers that are composed of hyaluronic acid in a clear gel form. Hyaluronic acid is a natural substance that has been synthesized to be safe, nonallergenic, and completely degradable, so there's no need for pretesting.

Allergic reactions are extremely rare. Restylane and Perlane are used to eliminate the following signs of aging:

- Wrinkles, furrows, and frown lines
- Pitting, scarring, and other surface damage to the skin
- Loss of fullness, particularly in the lips

How Do Restylane and Perlane Work?

The hyaluronic acid in both Restylane and Perlane is a nonanimal, stabilized hyaluronic acid (NASHA) in a clear, injectable gel form. Although your body naturally produces hyaluronic acid, this type is synthesized to be entirely free of animal proteins, which significantly reduces the possibility of allergic reactions.

The procedure for Restylane and Perlane injections is similar to that for collagen. Before treatment, an anesthetic may be applied, followed by a series of shallow injections with a very

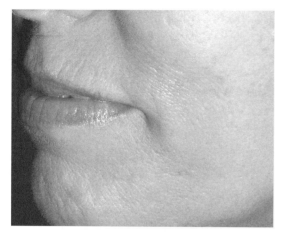

Lips before Restylane

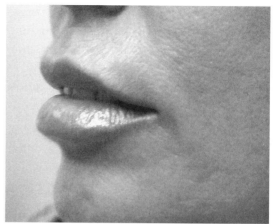

Lips after Restylane

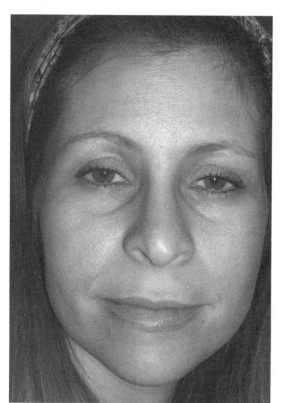

Tear troughs before Restylane

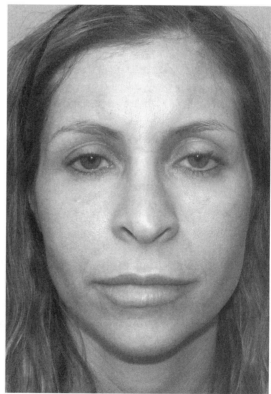

Tear troughs after Restylane

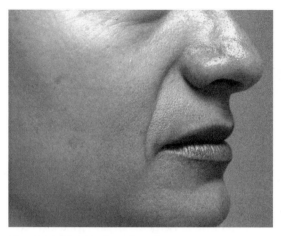
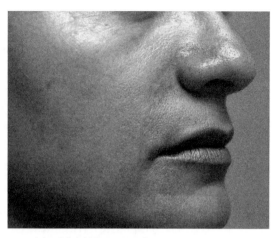

Nasolabial fold before Restylane   Nasolabial fold after Restylane

small needle, smoothing and filling out your specific problem areas. Injectable Restylane and Perlane treatments replenish your skin naturally, filling in depressions and augmenting soft-tissue features to give you a fresh, glowing, youthful look.

How Long Will Restylane and Perlane Last?

The average Restylane or Perlane treatment lasts six months. In the lower eyelid and nose regions, however, both products can last as long as twelve months. As with other fillers, the look is natural and immediate. The only difference among the fillers is duration and cost; they all look great the moment you walk out the door. If you need immediate gratification, that vibrant "wow" factor, there is only one procedure in cosmetic enhancement, and that is fillers.

Juvéderm

Juvéderm is another product that, like Restylane and Perlane, is composed of hyaluronic acid; it comes in the form of a gel that is injected into the skin. Juvéderm ULTRA, which is a mixture of Juvéderm and lidocaine, is pending approval by the FDA.

How Does Juvéderm Work?

Juvéderm is a smooth gel that flows into the skin; it was designed so that the overall effect would be smooth and natural rather than harsh and abrasive. In reality, Juvéderm is probably not that much different in effect or duration than Restylane or Perlane. Most physicians end up gravitating either to the Juvéderm or the Restylane/Perlane family.

How Many Times Must I Be Treated?

You must be treated about twice per year. Consult with your doctor after your first treatment to know how soon is too soon—or how long is too long—to go between treatments.

Are There Side Effects With Juvéderm?

As with all fillers, you can get temporary bruising, swelling and irregularity. You can also get nodule formation and a Tyndall effect with Juvéderm, as with Restylane.

How Long Will Juvéderm Last?

Although the manufacturer has been permitted by the FDA to claim twelve months' duration, the majority of people have to be re-treated in about six months. Similar to Restylane and Perlane, the product lasts longer in areas that have limited mobility, such as the lower eyelids and the nose.

Fascian

Fascian is an injectable human implant material that is made from the fascia, or the body's connective tissue. While Fascian treatments are still being performed, availability of the product for future use will be very limited.

How Does Fascian Work?

The active ingredient in Fascian is fascia lata from the covering of the abdominal muscle. Fascian implants have been used less frequently since other fillers have appeared. Their best use is for cheek augmentation.

How Many Times Must I Be Treated?

Most individuals subscribe to a regimen of three treatments in six months. Additional treatments can be administered as touch-ups once or twice during the remaining six months of the year.

Are There Side Effects with Fascian?

Concern remains that disease could be transmitted through human tissue although no proof exists that this is so. As with other fillers, you can get temporary bruising, swelling, and irregularity with Fascian.

How Long Will Fascian Last?

Fascian's duration is variable, but it lasts at least three months.

A (Slightly) Longer Story: More Than Twelve Months

Beauty takes time. Some procedures offer more duration than others and, as a result, require a commitment to a long-term regimen. In this section we discuss the following six procedures:

- Sculptra
- Fat (yes, fat!)
- Radiesse
- ArteFill
- Silicone

Sculptra

Sculptra (marketed outside the United States as New-Fill) is an injectable compound of poly-L-lactic (PLLA) acid gel. A synthetic polymer, Sculptra is designed to restore facial volume to areas of hollowness.

Sculptra is currently approved for use in people with lipoatrophy as a secondary aspect of HIV-related treatment and is pending FDA approval as Sculptra Cosmetic. Since its approval in 2004, the majority of its use has been off-label for aesthetic enhancements. The product works extremely well for individuals with moderate to severe volume loss. It is also extremely useful for areas such as the temples, the cheeks, the jawline, and around the mouth.

How Does Sculptra Work?

Sculptra works by encouraging new collagen growth and the formation of fibrous tissues that make the complexion look smooth, supple, and youthful after the initial filling effect has worn off. Sculptra provides a natural framework for your own soft-tissue growth and collagen production, creating natural volume and contour just where you want it. It is injected beneath the skin in a simple office procedure. The areas that are best treated by Sculptra are the cheeks, the jawline, and the temples. Sculptra primarily restores facial volume in a very natural and long-lasting manner. The lower eyelid region should be avoided except by very experienced injectors. The lips should never be treated with Sculptra.

How Many Times Must I Be Treated?

Generally speaking, most people require three to four treatments spaced one to two months apart. Up to five treatments may be necessary for individuals with severe facial volume loss.

Sculptra comes in a powder form and is mixed with water and lidocaine. As a result, patients have a very favorable experience due to the anesthetic solution.

Are There Side Effects with Sculptra?

Sculptra's safety has significantly improved over the past several years due to a refinement in injection techniques and treatment protocols. The main risks of Sculptra include bruising at the site of injection, nodule formation, and asymmetry. The overall risk of serious complications is well below 1 percent in the hands of an experienced physician. In fact, the company has a very comprehensive training protocol for injectors and only allows board-certified specialists to utilize the product. Special care should be taken if your practitioner recommends Sculptra for use under the eyes. Make sure that he or she has extensive experience using the product in that region.

How Long Will Sculptra Last?

The results from Sculptra can last for two years or longer. In our experience, most patients require a touch-up procedure between the second and third year. This is the key advantage of the product over other short-term fillers such as hyaluronic acids.

Radiesse

Radiesse is composed of calcium hydroxylapatite, a naturally occurring component found in the bones and the teeth that appears to have virtually no risk of allergic reaction when used as an implant. Radiesse has been used for many years for voice disorders.

How Does Radiesse Work?

Radiesse is injected with a small-gauge needle after the application of a topical anesthetic cream. Radiesse appears to have some biostimulatory effect that increases collagen production in the body. Radiesse was approved by the FDA for facial use in 2006, but many of us have been using it off-label for that purpose since 2001. We typically utilized Radiesse in the cheeks, the nasolabial folds, the jawline, and the hands. Its use has been improved over the past year as many practitioners have started adding a small amount of lidocaine to the syringe making it less painful and easier to inject. The eyelids and lips should be avoided. The photos at the top of page 120 show an actual patient of Dr. Hamilton's whose nasolabial folds have been treated.

The photos at the bottom of page 120 show an actual patient of Dr. Hamilton's whose cheek lines have been treated.

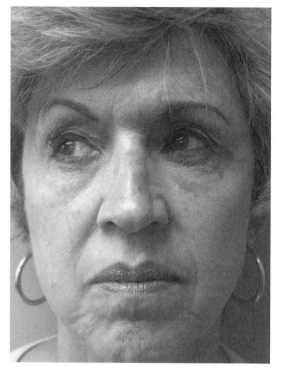

Before Radiesse

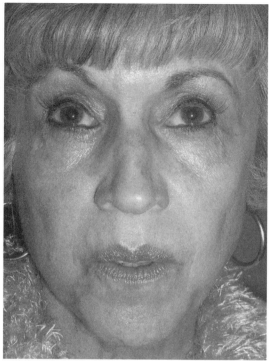

After Radiesse

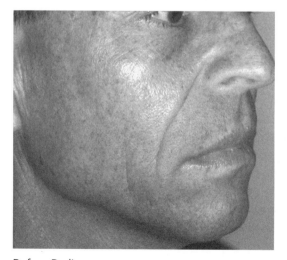

Before Radiesse

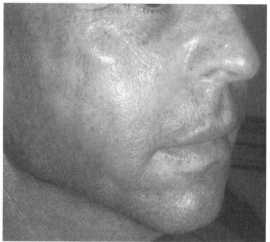

After Radiesse

How Many Times Must I Be Treated?

You will see your results on the day of the procedure. An initial treatment is generally augmented by a second session in one month. With the lidocaine mixture, the product is very well tolerated as compared to hyaluronic acids.

How Long Will Radiesse Last?

The effects last approximately one year.

ArteFill

Composed of polymethyl methacrylate (PMMA), lidocaine, and bovine collagen, ArteFill can permanently eliminate expression furrows: "smile lines," "marionette lines," brow and deep forehead lines, and depressed acne scars. The results look and feel extremely natural, since 80 percent of the fill is the patient's own collagen, produced over several months as a stimulation of the PMMA; the other 20 percent of the fill is the permanent PMMA microspheres themselves. Dr. Hamilton treated the first group of patients in the U.S. in 1997 and has been an FDA investigator for the product in two clinical trials. As of this writing, ArteFill distribution to physicians has been temporarilty halted due to company restructuring.

How Is ArteFill Administered?

The area to be treated is injected with ArteFill after the application of a topical anesthetic. Unlike prior approaches, such as collagen injections, ArteFill should not overcorrect the area (raise it up above flat skin level). There is immediate improvement because the area treated is raised to about normal skin level.

Is Allergy Testing Required for ArteFill?

You will have to be tested for an allergy to the collagen component of ArteFill by receiving a forearm injection and then wait one month to confirm that you are not allergic.

How Does ArteFill Work?

ArteFill injections include bovine collagen in addition to **PMMA**. As the collagen disappears in one to three months, the patient's own (permanent) collagen is produced more or less simultaneously to replace it. Studies have shown that the patient's collagen replaces most of the injected collagen, so most of the initial resolution of the wrinkle (or whatever is being treated) is permanent. The prevailing theory is that the patient's collagen has been stimulated by PMMA. Generally, there is minimal discomfort during ArteFill treatment, due to both the topical anesthetic and the lidocaine that is contained in the product.

How Many Times Must I Be Treated?

A minimum of two treatments is required, and you must wait at least three months between treatments. Sometimes one or two more treatments may be required. There is no maximum.

Are There Side Effects with ArteFill?

Rarely, as with almost any filler substance, inflammatory irregularities (small bumps) have been reported, but they are normally readily treatable. These allergic irregularities may occur anytime subsequent to the treatment (even years later).

If bumps do occur, they are generally quite small and are usually treated by injecting a cortisone-derived material into them. Based on follow-up data from an **FDA** trial, it appears that the chances of this occurring are considerably less than 1 percent. The manufacturing process is now performed in the United States, and it is expected that due to improved quality control, the incidences of these small irregularities will be reduced to negligible levels.

Can ArteFill Move?

No movement has been shown to occur, nor would it be expected to, because there really isn't anything to shift: PMMA droplets (microspheres of thirty to forty microns) are surrounded by the patient's own collagen and the microspheres are too large to be carried away by our cells.

Silicone

Silicone has a varied and checkered past, both in its injectable form and as a breast-implant device. It was widely misused as an injectable from the 1950s to the 1970s for augmentation of the breasts, penis, buttocks, lips, and face. It produced many instances of significant side effects, so its use was banned in the United States throughout the 1980s and 1990s. However, it has received renewed interest in the new millennium because it has become legally available again, being used off-label as a facial filler (its approved use is for the eye).

The most widely used form is Silikon 1000, which is medical grade and pure. Part of the reason for the side effects from silicone injections in earlier decades was undoubtedly contamination—both inadvertent and purposefully formulated—of the injectables; however, quantities, location of injection, injection experience, and individual allergies also played a role, though unknown issues remain.

Evaluation of the appropriateness of the variables (such as the quality and the frequency of treatment) in silicone augmentation of the face can be difficult, but one factor appears to be emerging: lip augmentation appears to be its best and safest use. Indeed, it is felt by many filler experts that silicone is the safest and most natural permanent filler augmentation product worldwide if administered through the microinjection microdroplet technique. This technique implants generally less than 1 cc of material into both lips. The use of silicone in other areas of the face appears to yield a much higher risk of allergic reaction (granulomas, or red bumps), which can occur years later.

How Does Silicone Work?

Silicone stimulates the production of collagen to enlarge the lips. Probably less than 1 percent of the enlargement is due to the silicone; the bulk is due to your own collagen. Two important issues should be noted:

1. The enlargement occurs gradually over months.
2. The feel is completely natural.

Silicone injections in the lips can be painful if they are done without an anesthetic. After a dental block injection in the mouth, however, there is essentially no discomfort at all. The dental block injection itself is painless due to the prior application of a topical anesthetic inside the mouth.

Are There Side Effects to Silicone?

The incidence of lumps or granulomas in silicone-treated lips appears to be close to negligible if the microdroplet technique is used.

Is Allergy Testing Required for Silicone?

Allergy testing is not required for silicone injections.

How Many Times Must I Be Treated?

Typically, three treatments are required, spaced three months apart.

Can Silicone Move?

Yes, there has been radiographic evidence of silicone migrating from its original injection location. The mechanism is poorly understood. This phenomenon has not been seen in the lip region.

Fat

Fat grafting utilizes your own body fat to augment facial volume loss. It is an outpatient procedure usually performed under local anesthesia that removes and refines fat tissues from the lower part of the body with liposuction. This refined fat is then injected into the multiple layers of the face with small needles, to restore facial volume. Live fat cells are transplanted near muscles that provide blood supply to the fat cells, which results in long-term transfer. We refer to it as *multilevel fat grafting* (MFG) because the fat is injected in multiple layers to improve its viability and increase overall appearance.

How Does MFG Work?

This procedure restores the facial volume loss that is associated with aging and with prior face-lifting procedures. Fat grafting significantly improves the skeletonization of the face, which is a hallmark of aging; thus, it restores a more youthful facial appearance. Fat grafting is often done simultaneously with a face-lift and blepharoplasty to produce a fuller and less flattening effect.

How Many Times Must I Be Treated?

Fat transfer has the potential of being a permanent procedure but may require two to three treatment session. In our experience 90 percent of the patients will obtain the desired results with one session. The procedure involves performing liposuction to harvest fat from the belly, the hips, or the thighs. The fat is then put in small syringes and then strategically reinjected to replace lost volume or reshape the face. Today's injection techniques allow doctors to place fat where significant amounts will survive. Fat is commonly injected in places such as the hollows under the eyes, the midface, the nasolabial folds, the lips, around the mouth, and around the jawline.

Are There Side Effects with MFG?

Fat grafting is a safe procedure that has been used for many years with good results. The overall complication rate is less than 1 percent in the hands of an experienced surgeon. The main risks are asymmetry, irregularity, overcorrection, undercorrection, and the need for repeat treatments.

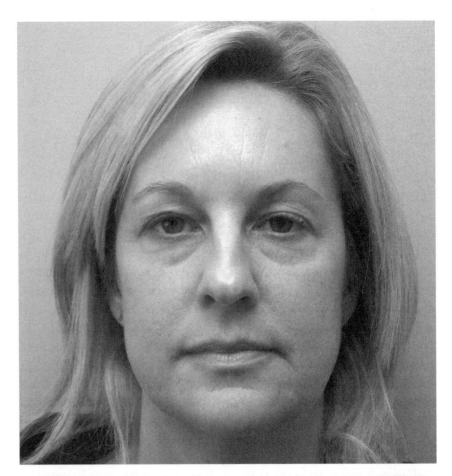

Face before MFG
and blepharoplasty

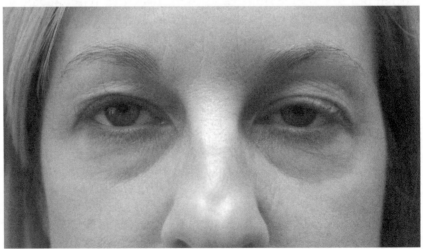

Eyes before MFG
and blepharoplasty

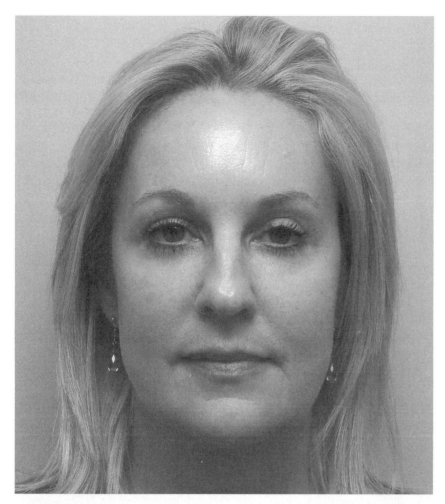

Face after MFG
and blepharoplasty

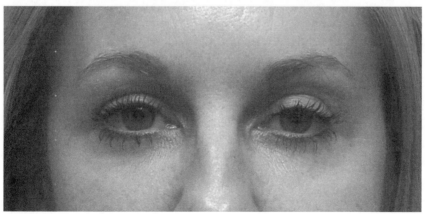

Eyes after MFG
and blepharoplasty

WHAT YOUR FACIAL PLASTIC SURGEON OR DERMATOLOGIST CAN AND CANNOT DO FOR YOU

As much as we'd like to be miracle workers, we are not. There are things we simply can and cannot do. Modern technology is great, but we are a long way away from performing a face transplant as a lunch-time aging fix, no matter what Hollywood—our closest neighbor—might have you think!

The Top Five Things Your Facial Plastic Surgeon or Dermatologist *Can* Do for You

There is plenty that we *can* do to make you look and feel years younger today. We can do the following:

1. Shave years off your chronological age by combining various products and procedures that are right for you
2. Make you feel young, glamorous, sexy, and beautiful again
3. Work with you to create a lifelong plan for facial rejuvenation
4. Talk you out of expensive and intensive procedures that are wrong for you and into less severe but more effective procedures that are right for you
5. Give you your confidence back

The Top Five Things Your Plastic Surgeon or Dermatologist *Cannot* Do for You

Every day, people walk through our doors asking for the impossible. Whether it's a misconception about the results of some new procedure or simply the hope that a nip and a tuck can take thirty, instead of ten, years off your appearance, it just isn't possible—and we can do only what's possible.

So before you even ask, here is our list of the top five things a plastic surgeon or dermatologist *cannot* do for you:

1. Put a celebrity's nose on your face
2. Put a celebrity's head on your body
3. Make you a celebrity just by changing your appearance
4. Introduce you to Jessica Alba or Ben Affleck
5. Get you courtside tickets to a Lakers game

How Long Will MFG Last?

In 90 percent of people, fat grafting will have a sustained, long-lasting result. Ten percent of individuals will require repeat injections over a period of several months. As with any other fillers, the aging process will continue even with permanent transfer.

7

The Face-Lift Alternatives

Tightening Devices and Volume Restoration

Before Botox, Restylane, and Thermage and all the lotions, potions, lasers, products, and procedures we've catalogued throughout this book, the default term for any surgical cosmetic procedure for the last few decades was pretty much this: *face-lift*. "Tight was right," and having as few as possible wasn't even an issue; more were better and, quite often, not good enough. You would commonly hear questions and comments such as the following:

"When are you getting a face-lift?"

"Did you see Maryanne's new face-lift?"

"The plastic surgeon said I needed a face-lift."

"Do you think I need a face-lift?"

"How soon before I can get another face-lift?"

Questions like these and so many more were popular fare at water coolers, gyms, fundraisers, and PTA luncheons throughout the land, and without any other clear options, face-lifts became the be-all and end-all of plastic surgery.

How times have changed. Today there are so many other non-surgical options and so much patient- and doctor-driven education to inform people about the various surgical procedures that now exist that most of us realize there are many steps on the way to a face-lift. Furthermore, a face-lift itself is not the inevitable solution to fixing what you want to change. This chapter is designed to help you discover what the alternatives are and, more important, where you fit on the "do I 'need' a face-lift" scale. We will teach you a new scale that doesn't necessarily involve how old you are or what you think you need.

Age is not, we emphasize, the determining factor in whether you "need" a face-lift. In our practices we've both learned that age is not the indicator. Both of us know dozens of individuals in their fifties who have no reason to have a face-lift—and just as many in their forties who do.

Where do you fall on this scale? To determine the answer, we must consider the two mitigating factors that we will discuss in this chapter:

1. **Laxity.** As we have discussed, *laxity* is our term for looseness and sagginess, otherwise known as drooping.
2. **Volume loss.** As your skin ages, it loses volume and becomes more brittle and less supple, creating a more gaunt look to the face.

How much laxity and volume loss you have on a scale—mild to moderate, or moderate to severe—can help your doctor to determine whether you should have a face-lift. It's vital that you know beforehand, so that you can come to your doctor as prepared as possible.

This chapter and the next are designed to help you discover what nonsurgical procedures are right for you and, if necessary, what nonsurgical procedures might be complementary to any surgical procedures your physician might recommend. Gone are the days of one procedure fits all.

Today, most doctors customize a diagnosis that is based not just on the degree of laxity and volume loss but also on the patient's specific personality, pain and recovery threshold, and a variety of other factors. To perfectly tailor your procedure, or combination of procedures, you and your doctor should work together as two equal parts of your own personal doctor-patient team.

That is why it is so important for you to be educated before you speak with your physician; being intimidated by all those degrees on the wall behind his or her head is no way to feel on an equal footing with your doctor.

You want to be able to discuss your options, openly and honestly, without any fear that you are asking "dumb" questions and with the knowledge that your physician is interested in the unique and personal you. A generic diagnosis won't do here; it has to be personal and unique to you and your specific needs if you are to get the results you desire.

A lot of what we do with our patients is actually trying to undo what the popular media and decades of hearing *face-lift* have already done to them. Many people think that a face-lift is the ultimate in plastic surgery or the gold standard of surgical procedures; others think that all of the creams and lotions and skin care are things you use until the inevitable aging process makes a face-lift equally inevitable.

This is not true; as we always say in our offices, the best procedure is the one you avoid by taking care of your skin in the first place. Just as important, through a complement of various surgical and nonsurgical procedures, you can avoid a face-lift altogether—at least for the time being.

Then again, perhaps the years have been unkind to you, and because of that, in addition to your genetics, the option of a face-lift makes more sense; so be it. Chapter 8 will cover all that—and then some. In this chapter we are focusing on people with the early laxity and volume loss that a typical face-lift isn't going to fix.

A face-lift too soon is only going to make matters worse in later years, just as waiting too long is going to make the option of a face-lift later just that much more imperative. The key is to know what to do and when; we're here to help you do just that.

The two issues we'll be talking about in this chapter are:

- **Tightening.** Modern physicians do a balancing act of helping people to achieve skin that is not too loose or too tight but just right. When we say *tightening*, we are not talking about a too-tight, harsh look that is the result of going to one extreme to avoid the other. Our main goal in restoring youth to an aging face is to recapture the full, supple look of youth; that is why we don't want to mislead or misdirect you into seeking a treatment that tightens too much—or not enough.

- **Volume restoration.** The current medical philosophy is that the aging process does not involve just laxity; volume loss also comes into play. The best way to think about how volume loss affects your face is to picture a man who weighs 250 pounds. He wears his best suit, which fits perfectly, to the doctor's office, where his family physician tells him that he must lose fifty pounds. Six months later, after having made a New Year's resolution to lose fifty pounds, the same man steps on the scale to find success: he weighs two hundred pounds! Once again he puts on his favorite suit to go see his doctor, but he's got a problem: the suit is too loose. It hangs and sags and bags and droops in all the wrong places. This is how the aging process affects your face; the skin we have becomes too big for the bones we have, so it sags and hangs over. By restoring volume, we help you to "fit" into your face again; there are a variety of products and procedures to help you do that.

Of course, every patient is unique. Some have laxity but not volume loss; some have volume loss but no laxity. Others have both. The following are the variables that we most typically see in our offices:

- **People who have a little bit of laxity and not a lot of volume loss.** Perhaps you've noticed places where your skin hangs loosely, drags, or even bags, but you and your doctor both realize that in most respects your face has the fullness and suppleness that makes it still look youthful.
- **People who have a little bit of volume loss and not a lot of laxity.** Perhaps your face is looking gaunt and hollow, and shadows are starting to form; it has lost volume, yet you don't have sagging or bagging issues.
- **People who have both volume loss and laxity.** As they age, some people experience both laxity and volume loss, so both must be addressed.

Which category applies to you? Don't worry if you can't answer just yet. By the end of this chapter, you will know exactly which category you fall into and, best of all, which product or procedure can help you to correct it.

The Grape versus the Pea: Youthful Does Not Equal Tight

The trouble with treating a face-lift as the default, mandatory procedure for all things aging is that there are many misconceptions about what exactly a face-lift is.

The generic face-lift simply pulls back the features of the face until they are tight or flat, creating a two-dimensional windswept effect. Many people don't see the problem with this because they've been taught by the popular media (television or fashion magazines) that "tight equals youthful," so naturally they desire that tight and flat effect. As we've already mentioned, however, it's extremely important to become aware of your misconceptions and not be surprised if you learn something new along the way.

In this case, we have to tell you that tight does *not* equal youthful; it simply equals tight. The attractiveness of youthful skin comes from its fullness and its suppleness—not its tight, brittle nature, which is an effect that increases with age. Thus, you do not want to simply get a two-dimensional, one-size-fits-all face-lift that simply pulls the skin back tighter and flatter across your face.

We always recommend a "three-dimensional face-lift," which, despite its name, is not always a surgical face-lift. We frequently recommend multilevel fat grafting (MFG, which we discussed in the previous chapter) to create the three-dimensional effect; at other times, a procedure known as the *liquid face-lift* (which we discuss below) is recommended. For individuals with moderate to severe laxity, a surgical three-dimensional face-lift is performed where MFG, fillers, and/or implants are combined with a customized face-lift (this will be discussed in later chapters in detail). This tactic allows us to address the underlying cause of aging rather than just camouflaging the aging process.

How does a three-dimensional face-lift beat the two-dimensional version? It might help you to revisit the grape and raisin metaphor we used earlier: A youthful, healthy, radiant face is like a grape—fresh, juicy, and firm. As we age, however, facial volume loss creates a more raisinlike effect; the face flattens and shrinks to become brittle and allow for wrinkles, sagging, and bagging.

Now we want you to ponder a new question: What would you rather have as the result of your face-lift—a pea or a grape? Think carefully before you answer. A two-dimensional, cookie-cutter face-lift merely peels back the skin of the raisin to make it even more tight and flat than it already is. You don't get a "grape" at all; what you get in this instance is a tighter, smaller surface area that more closely resembles a pea.

What a three-dimensional, or liquid, face-lift does is to reinflate the "raisin" rather than peel it back or flatten it out; it reinjects new life into it. It gives you the sense of fullness, firmness, and youthfulness that you desire in a procedure; your skin gets back the tone and feel of a grape, not a pea.

Tightening Devices for Dealing with Mild to Moderate Laxity

If your pants become loose, you simply tighten your belt, right? The problem is solved. Well, your face should be no different. Although it may sound simplistic, the procedures are so numerous and so advanced these days that it really is no more difficult than that for a qualified medical physician.

If the procedures are performed properly in a medical setting by a trained professional, the risk and downtime involved with any of them is very, very low. Most are outpatient procedures with little downtime and with results that will impress you. If you have only mild to moderate laxity, therefore, you are in luck: not only is a face-lift not a good option for you now; if you continue practicing good skin care and avail yourself of several nonsurgical procedures, you might be able to delay more invasive procedures for the forseeable future.

We will deal first with tightening devices, which address only the issue of laxity. In the next section we will handle the second critical issue, volume loss, by recommending several products and procedures that restore volume to the aging face.

In this section we discuss the following four tightening devices for dealing with mild to moderate laxity:

* Thermage
* Titan
* ReFirme
* Accent

Although these are the four most popular procedures, by no means are they created equal, and we will take great pains to differentiate them for you and highlight each one's pros and cons. None of these four treatments requires surgery.

Thermage

Thermage is the most commonly used safe and effective treatment for moderate laxity (or looseness of facial skin or flesh). In our opinion, Thermage is the gold standard for tightening devices.

Thermage is safe and noninvasive, requires no downtime, and is applied in a single treatment. It works by heating the skin to over 61 degrees Celsius (thermal heating). This induces contraction of collagen which produces a tightening effect over a period of six months. Some tightening is noted on the day of the procedure, with gradual improvement over the next several months. Additionally, there is new collagen production in the dermis (the thick part of the skin). Thermage is clinically proven to tighten, contour, and rejuvenate facial skin to help naturally restore a more youthful appearance. (Used above the eyes, Botox can also be extremely helpful for firming up loose skin.)

When Thermage first came into use six or seven years ago, the protocol used resulted in only a 30 percent satisfaction rate. Today, with a change in the treatment protocol algorithm, accompanied by less pain, lower energy, and slightly longer

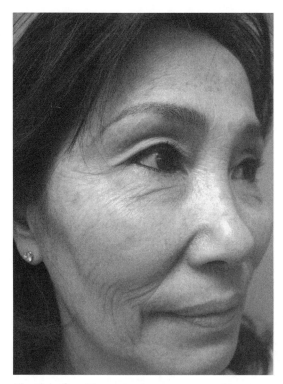

Cheek before Thermage

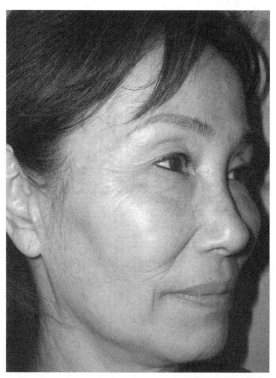

Cheek three months after Thermage

treatment time, Thermage's unique capacitive radio-frequency (CRF) technology yields a satisfaction rate of more than 92 percent in several reports.

Titan

Titan purports to have similar features as Thermage, particularly in its claims of "deep dermal heating with new collagen formation over time." Titan uses infrared light to heat the skin of the face. The depth of skin heating is less than occurs with Thermage and, therefore, the tightening effects may be less pronounced. Thermal heating that extends deep into the skin is associated with the production of more collagen, which helps to tighten and firm the face.

Christine Lee, a well-known dermatologist, did a split-face study and reported that it could take approximately three Titan treatments to equal one Thermage treatment. Once again, the expertise of the physician who is providing the procedure plays a crucial role in how safe and effective the procedure will be.

WORST-CASE SCENARIOS: WHEN PLASTIC SURGERY GOES WRONG

We have seen some pretty bad attempts at facial rejuvenation over the years. We have seen noses cut too severely, skin burned by faulty laser devices or inexperienced handlers, hair removal that backfired, and botched breast, chest, chin, and buttocks implants. Fortunately, these circumstances are extremely rare in the hands of an experienced and qualified physician.

We encourage you to make sure that your physician is qualified to perform the procedure or surgery that he or she recommends. Avoid price shopping for cosmetic surgery. Make sure that you ask all the right questions, and if your gut instinct tells you that the procedure or the surgeon does not make sense, then seek a second or even a third opinion.

If you do have a major complication, you should seek the advice of an experienced surgeon who specializes in revisional surgery.

ReFirme

Another skin-tightening procedure that is very popular on the market today is ReFirme. Like the other tightening procedures, ReFirme addresses the common signs of aging, including sagginess under the eyes, saggy brow lines, jowls and neck laxity, and nasolabial folds.

Using a combination of bipolar radio-frequency and light energies, ReFirme heats the dermal tissue to treat the affected area and go deep below the dermal layers to manipulate the collagen beneath the skin. Unlike conventional lasers and intense pulsed light, ReFirme uses significantly less optical energy, ensuring enhanced safety and a virtually painless procedure.

Accent

Accent is another radio-frequency device that is used to tighten the skin and reduce the effects of aging. Accent's radio-frequency treatments can create dramatic change without requiring invasive surgery or even topical anesthetics.

Accent is designed to uniformly heat the dermis with radio-frequency energy while protecting the epidermis with built-in contact cooling. The increased temperature in the dermis causes collagen contraction, realignment, and new collagen production, which continues to build over several months.

Volume Restoration for a Full, Youthful Look

In this section we will focus primarily on the following two treatments, which are both safe and effective face-lift alternatives:

- **The liquid face-lift.** For mild to moderate amounts of aging changes and volume loss, this procedure works very well. Utilizing products like Radiesse and Sculptra to correct signs of volume loss, the physician injects the midface and lower face with a liquid filler, hence the name *liquid face-lift*.

- **Multilevel fat grafting.** For mild to moderate volume loss, multilevel fat grafting (MFG) has really revolutionized how we look at a face. A lot of our patients used to get face-lifts, but they didn't look right because it was too much procedure for what was actually required to fix the problem. The patient needed volume restoration, not tightening or flattening; the patient needed three-dimensional rather than two-dimensional. Fat grafting is a one-hour procedure, done under local anesthesia at the doctor's office, in which the physician simply harvests some fat from the belly, the hips, or the thighs and then separates out the fat cells and injects them into the desired areas of the face—below the skin and above the muscle—to create a fuller, more youthful effect.

You will not read about this material in many other current books on facial rejuvenation, skin care, or aging, because what we're suggesting is truly a paradigm shift from the days when face-lifts ruled supreme and were done almost exclusively to treat any and all aging issues of the face.

We suggest that you cast away what you thought you knew about face-lifts and open yourself up to the information we're presenting here. Furthermore, be open to discussing these procedures with your doctor. (There will be more on how to choose a doctor in chapter 10.)

This information is not absolute; it is informative. In other words, we can't diagnose you through the pages of this book as having mild to moderate laxity and/or volume loss. You might have more than that—or even less. That is why your physician must be chosen carefully, so that you both have an easy and comfortable flow of information.

We also suggest that you be open to treating tightening and volume loss as complementary, not exclusive, products and procedures. Perhaps you could use treatment for both tightening *and* volume loss; in that case, a Thermage treatment might be complemented by MFG or even a liquid face-lift.

> *You will not read about this material in many other current books on facial rejuvenation, skin care, or aging, because what we're suggesting is truly a paradigm shift from the days when face-lifts ruled supreme and were done almost exclusively to treat any and all aging issues of the face.*

This is not about your doctor simply trying to pump up your bill; it is about your physician trying to give you the effect you truly desire, using the variety and volume of procedures that are currently on the market. Even when we do surgical face-lifts, we often complement them with MFG or fillers, to avoid a tight, flat, windswept look and to increase volume and fullness for a more natural, youthful effect.

It's no different from going to the dentist and getting a whitening treatment to complement your recent cleaning or, for that matter, going to the garage and getting an oil change plus a tune-up for your car; the two services complement each other for results that you couldn't get by using just one.

The Liquid Face-Lift: "Filling" the Void between Surgical and Nonsurgical Alternatives

As we have seen throughout this book, four major components of the facial structure change as one ages: skin, fat, muscle, and bone. Loss of elasticity in the skin and soft tissues, loss of volume, reabsorption of the bone, and gravity's effects (sagging) are all signs of aging. In this chapter we have concerned ourselves with two primary culprits: volume loss and laxity.

Why are there so many alternatives to a face-lift? It's not because we're against face-lifts—that's for sure. However, it's time to shift our perspective from the face-lift as cure-all to the face-lift as a complement to several other viable, safe, and healthy alternatives. It's also time to stop thinking of the face-lift as the gold standard of facial rejuvenation; it's simply not.

For example, a face-lift does not solve all of the problems of aging, such as age spots and/or surface texture changes, nor does it create a three-dimensional, fuller, firmer, youthful effect—unless it's complemented by various alternative measures that we've discussed throughout this chapter (and will discuss further in chapter 8).

Very few procedures have wide-ranging results; most are specialized treatments for a particular problem, such as volume loss or laxity. Fortunately, a variety of techniques is now available to help with the aging process.

For instance, various degrees of wrinkles and folds on different areas of the face can be addressed with the use of injectables in a face-lift procedure. Plumping up facial volume and filling furrows (deep wrinkles) can be addressed by using dermal fillers. Expression-related creases are caused by muscle contractions; however, with the use of muscle-relaxing agents such as Botox, these creases can be softened and made to appear more youthful on the forehead and around the eyes.

Injectables, which are the main materials used in a liquid face-lift, can address the following:

- Lost fullness
- Expression lines
- Flattened or hollowed features

After an examination, you and your physician should draw up a treatment plan that is designed specifically for the signs of aging and your personal goals. This is a critical phase, and we strongly urge you to use all of the information, power, and confidence you've gained while reading this book to go into your initial consultation as prepared as possible.

What kinds of injectables are used in a liquid face-lift? Generally longer-lasting injectables like Radiesse, Sculptra, and ArteFill are combined with Botox, hyaluronic acids, and collagen.

Injecting fillers at various depths to fill creases creates a more youthful contour and appearance. Treatment can take as little as thirty minutes, depending on the number of injection sites and the injectables that are used. Restylane and Juvéderm fill lips and tear-trough areas under the eyes while collagen products fill fine lines and thinner tissues. Radiesse and Sculptra create new curve, fill deep crevices, and restore lost volume. Botox softens expression lines.

Injectable face-lift results are usually visible instantly; however, if Sculptra is used, it can take up to three sessions to see improvement. Sessions are spaced about a month apart, with improvement occurring gradually.

It is common to have multiple injection sites, and swelling and bruising may be experienced the first few days after treatment. To minimize swelling, patients leave the office with a pack of ice and are advised not to exercise for the first few hours in order to prevent an increase in heart rate or blood pressure. It is helpful (though not essential) for patients to avoid vitamin E, anti-inflammatories, fish oil, and any blood-thinning medications (aspirin and ibuprofen) that promote bruising.

The duration depends on which fillers were used in the liquid face-lift procedure. Collagen-based fillers last three to four months, hyaluronic acid–based fillers can last from six to twelve months, and semipermanent injectables (Radiesse, Sculptra) can last one to two years or more. Botox lasts from three to four months and may help temporary fillers to last longer by decreasing muscle action. In order to fine-tune the results, follow-up treatments may be necessary.

As you read this chapter, remember that it applies just to *early to moderate* volume loss and laxity at the onset of aging. If your laxity and/or volume loss is *moderate to severe*, you will find greater relief in the following chapter on surgical alternatives.

It is important, however, to read both chapters to inform yourself on what alternatives exist on the market today and for whom they are intended. Fillers, injectables, and MFG may be enough to restore early to moderate signs of aging but not enough to conquer moderate to more severe laxity. Once you get past a certain point, you may require a surgical facial rejuvenation procedure such as blepharoplasty, endoscopic browlifts, and/or customized face-lift procedures.

The case for using popular, safe, and effective injectables to achieve a liquid face-lift is strong, but remember that it all depends on the initial analysis with your doctor. Be clear about your expectations and discuss all alternatives, openly and honestly, with your physician.

Rest assured, there are many instances where a surgical face-lift is warranted; the next chapter is all about surgical face-lifts and their many benefits. However, a qualified physician should tell you about all the available alternatives during your initial consultation, and if he or she doesn't, it is your responsibility to ask.

Now that you know that there is a difference between mild to moderate and moderate to severe laxity and volume loss, you can be more educated about which products and procedures are right for you. This shouldn't threaten your physician or make him or her defensive; we love it when people come to us prepared, because it makes for a more open and productive initial consultation.

Many people are nervous during the initial consultation, and with good reason. Here is a doctor showing you "the future you" on a computer monitor, measuring and adjusting and marking your face, and if you don't have an open mind, the experience can seem genuinely negative; this is someone who is basically pointing out or reminding you of your physical "flaws." You must be open and honest about your expectations and needs and require the same openness and honesty from your doctor.

What you want and what you require can be two different things; we have an ethical responsibility to point out to a patient when there is a difference. You might want Thermage and not a face-lift, for instance, when the results you want actually require a face-lift and not Thermage.

The converse is equally true; we often recommend less than a face-lift if it's not required. Years ago, most physicians simply gave everyone a face-lift who asked for one; today we are in an advanced era, and don't need to use the scalpel each time, especially not when a filler or an injectable will do.

Prevention is still the best cure, and not just in how you take care of your skin on a daily basis. What you do *before* a procedure is just as important as what happens *during* the procedure and how you care for yourself *after* the procedure.

It all comes down to the initial facial analysis performed by your skin-care professional; you have to know what the problem is so that the right solution presents itself. Someone who has pure volume loss doesn't need Thermage; someone who has good volume and just some laxity doesn't need volume restoration. Meanwhile, someone with volume loss and laxity requires a combination of products and procedures to address both concerns for the desired results.

Who Said Fat Is Bad for You? A Guide to Multilevel Fat Grafting

If this were a diet book, we might not be writing this section, particularly not with the above heading. In our practices, however, fat is *good* news, not bad. That's because there is now a fattening procedure to make a person look young. The procedure, multilevel fat grafting (MFG), was described in chapter 6. It plumps up the face by injecting fat that has been harvested from the belly, the hips, or the thighs—areas where fat is usually plentiful.

MFG is a new noninvasive restorative approach to aesthetic surgery that facilitates the enhancement of facial volume to provide a more youthful appearance. We often utilize MFG simultaneously with face-lifts and blepharoplasty to improve the overall results.

Procedure Highlights

* Pure fat cells are taken from the abdomen, the hips, or the thighs of the patient.
* The live fat cells are injected into layers of the face.
* These cells age along with the normal facial fat cells.
* Almost 90 percent of the people who have the procedure get successful results in the first try.
* Others (about 10 percent) may require two or three procedures to achieve full correction.
* The transferred fat incorporates permanently into the

face; the aging process continues, however, so you are not completely out of the woods. Most patients will typically follow-up in five years to re-evaluate their facial appearance.

Procedure Disadvantages

- There may be some swelling and bruising, but this disappears in a week. Subtle swelling may take several weeks to subside.
- It is not recommended for people with kidney or liver disease or who have very little body fat.

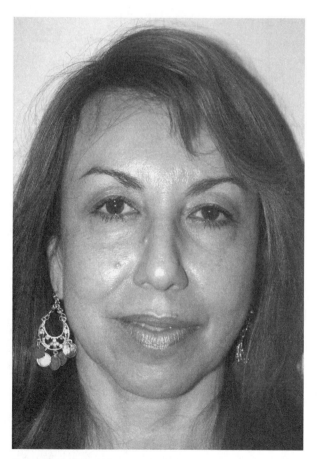

Before face-lift with MFG, front view

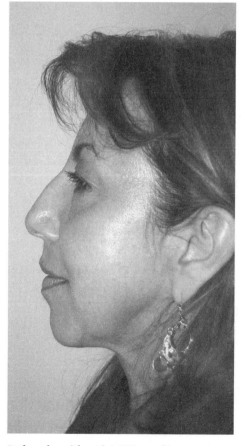

Before face-lift with MFG, profile

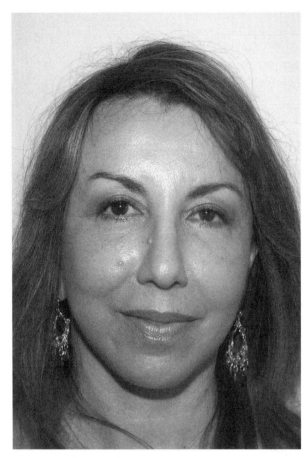

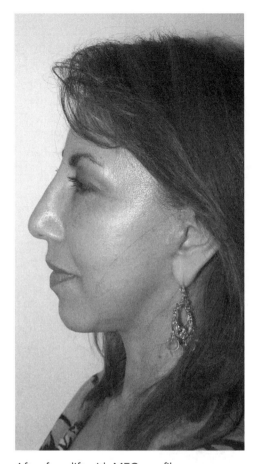

After face-lift with MFG, front view   After face-lift with MFG, profile

The Eyes Have It: Nonsurgical Alternatives to the Eyelid Lift

Throughout this section we have been primarily concerned with laxity and volume loss, but what about treating such sensitive areas as the eyes? Rest assured that as the face goes, so go the eyes; today there is a variety of nonsurgical alternatives with which to treat this critical area, which is so vital to retaining your desired youthful appearance.

As the art and science of eyelid rejuvenation have advanced, there has been a significant improvement in the nonsurgical solutions for improving the appearance of the eyes. In the past decade we have learned that volume loss in and around the eyes contributes significantly to the aging process of the area.

As a result, we utilize nonsurgical volume restoration to address these areas in appropriate candidates. The main advance here is the use of in-office injectables to improve the hollowness of the area under the eyes and the laxity of the upper eyelids. The three products that are commonly employed in eyelid lifts are Restylane, Juvéderm, and fat.

As described in earlier chapters, Restylane and Juvéderm are hyaluronic acids (proteins that are naturally found in the skin). Restylane or Juvéderm is generally injected in the tear-trough region (or hollows) under the eyes and can also be used to reduce the laxity of the upper eyelids by improving the position of the eyebrows and restoring fullness to the sunken portions of the eyelids. Restylane and Juvéderm generally have few side effects, and their results can last up to twelve months in the tear-trough area. Hyaluronic acids should be injected deep to the muscle in order to avoid irregularities and bluish discoloration clinically referred to as the Tyndall effect.

Botox injections can also be used to reduce crow's feet and elevate the brows (chemical brow lift), further enhancing the overall appearance. MFG can achieve results similar to those of Restylane and Juvéderm. The main difference, however, is that fat transfer is usually a more long-term solution—and for about 90 percent of individuals, with just one injection. For individuals with significant hollowness and sagging, fat provides better results than hyaluronic products.

Is There Such a Thing as a Nonsurgical Nose Job?

Nose surgery is one of the most popular cosmetic procedures around, and it has been for years. In the past, rhinoplasty was the only available option for people who were looking to improve the

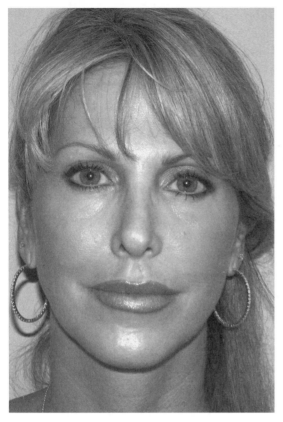

Before revision tip rhinoplasty

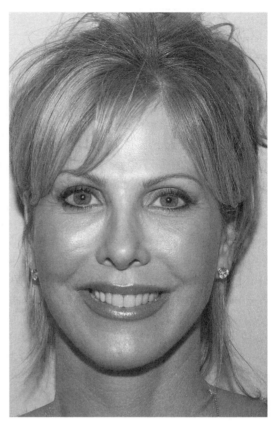

After revision tip rhinoplasty

size and shape of the nose. In the past few years, "nonsurgical rhinoplasty" has become popular. Hyaluronic acids, Radiesse, silicone, and ArteFill are being used by practitioners to fill depressions, smooth out sharp angles, or change the angle of the tip of the nose.

There can be significant complications from the misuse of injectables in the nose, especially in the hands of inexperienced practitioners. We have seen disastrous results when the procedure is performed by physicians who do not understand the aesthetics and anatomy of the nose.

We recommend utilizing fillers for minor corrections and avoiding a major overhaul of the nose. We prefer hyaluronic acids for this procedure since it is reversible and well tolerated in nasal skin. We have also used Radiesse with good success but with much more caution. We avoid using fillers in the patients who are planning on having a rhinoplasty procedure in the future as injectables can significantly interfere with surgical dissection.

Generally speaking, rhinoplasty specialists would be the ideal physicians to utilize fillers in the nasal region.

8

The Surgical Answers

Fixing Sagging Brows, Eyelids, Cheeks, and More

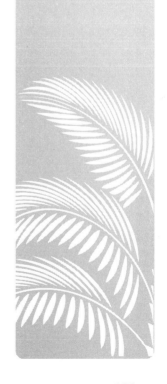

If you're worried about having facial plastic surgery, we want to put your fears to rest; modern medicine is so advanced that much of the risk that was experienced during former surgical procedures has become a thing of the past.

Don't get us wrong; risk exists with every surgical procedure, no matter how minor or major it appears on the surface. However, if you do your homework, trust your physician, are confident in his or her credentials, and have discussed the pros and cons of the procedure with your doctor, the chance of serious harm or injury is likely to be less than 1 percent. (Chapter 9 discusses how to further reduce even this small chance.)

Today, facial plastic surgery is being performed routinely in doctors' offices, surgical centers, and hospitals all across the country. We do not claim that nonsurgical procedures are more or less risky than surgical procedures; we only want to educate you on both types of procedures so that you will have a choice when discussing your own personal, unique needs with your physician. Nonsurgical and surgical procedures are like apples and oranges; they are very different but equally beneficial, depending on your personal wants and needs.

Although the focus of this chapter is facial plastic surgery, surgery is not the *only* answer today. Moreover, even when you have surgery, your doctors will still have to do maintenance work with fillers, lasers, lotions, and potions to keep you looking youthful years down the road.

That is why it is so critical to have a healthy, lasting, trusting relationship with your physician. To retain your youthful appearance, you will be seeing him or her several times in the next few years—and beyond—regardless of how little or how much plastic surgery you have had. Surgery is neither a cure-all nor a time machine; it won't bring you back to the luster and youth of your eighteen-year-old skin, and you will still have to maintain and take care of your skin once the surgery is over.

You have to take personal responsibility for your plastic surgery, no matter what procedure you're getting or, for that matter, who is performing it. This responsibility begins with information, and reading this book is a great place to start. Even more important, however, is to implement this book by going into your initial consultation armed with knowledge, confidence, and the right questions.

Finally, keep in mind that getting plastic surgery is a lot like doing a major renovation on your house. The roof, the garage door, or the swimming pool may be brand new, and the place looks great now, but that doesn't mean you can stop mowing the lawn or vacuuming the carpet. Your face is a living, breathing entity, and it is up to you and your surgeon to work together to put it—and keep it—in the best shape of your life. Proper skin care and routine maintenance are a big part of that, just as regular housekeeping and periodic touch-ups keep your house looking well kept and new.

There is a lot of ground to cover in this chapter, but that's good for you, because we guarantee that by the time you are through reading, you will know "everything you always wanted to know about facial plastic surgery but were afraid to ask." To divide this information into digestible pieces, we will highlight three sections of the face: the eyes and the surrounding area (the brow and the midface); the lower face and the neck; and the profile (the nose and the chin).

Diagrams of the facial regions involved, as well as "before" and "after" pictures of our own patients, should help to increase your understanding of each specific procedure.

When you go to see your doctor for a primary consultation, all regions of the face will be evaluated to achieve a balanced and aesthetically pleasing outcome. In much the same way, surgical and nonsurgical methods are often combined to get the optimum outcome. The following regions and surgical options will be discussed:

- **The eyes.** As we discussed earlier, the eyelids have two annoying "neighbors." The forehead and eyebrows are the "upstairs neighbor," and the midface and cheeks are the "downstairs neighbor." As a result, the evaluation of this region of the face includes how the brow, the eyes, and the transition from the lower eyelids to the midface work in concert with one another to create your current appearance—and what can be done about each to obtain your desired outcome. The surgical procedures that address these issues include the following:

    Blepharoplasty: plastic surgery of the eyes
    Brow lift: endoscopic forehead lift and other alternatives
    Endoscopic midface-lifts
    Multilevel fat grafting
    Cheek implants

- **The lower face and the neck.** The lower face encompasses the jawline and the underside of the chin; we also include the neck in this category, because the features of all three are very common in terms of a surgical procedure. The common procedures to address these sensitive areas include the following:

> Face-lift and neck lift (rhytidectomy)
> Multilevel fat grafting
> Chin implants

A DAY IN THE LIFE OF YOUR PLASTIC SURGEON OR DERMATOLOGIST

People often ask us what our days are like. Which celebrity did we see or work on today? How many movie premieres did we go to this week? How many rounds of golf did we play? Actually, be it in Beverly Hills or in your town, doctors are all the same: we are basically workaholics with a glamorous address.

Our days begin early as we pore over the latest updates, journals, or research reports before heading to the office for the day's first appointment. Once we greet our first patient, the race is on. If a surgical procedure or a celebrity client is going to take longer than expected or require special attention, we plan and schedule accordingly. To accommodate our demanding schedules, we like to keep our offices running smoothly and our appointments on time.

Although we might have one of the most glamorous addresses in the world, even celebrities want their work done quickly and quietly, with little fanfare. Since most of our A-list clientele prefer to keep our professional relationship private, we receive very few invitations to red carpet movie premieres or other A-list events. Sorry!

On the other hand, we do have fun working in Beverly Hills. We often walk down Rodeo or Bedford Drive and see world-famous actors, singers, and other 90210 doctors. There are always paparazzi around, and once in a while we see Paris Hilton ordering frozen yogurt next door.

Finally, no matter what our address is and where we live, we are physicians first and foremost. The Hippocratic Oath applies to aesthetic surgery, and we never forget that fact. We treat every individual as if he or she is a star who must get prepared for the red carpet. Everybody should be treated accordingly.

- **The profile.** Your profile encompasses both your nose and your chin, which become more prominent when viewed from the side. The common surgical procedures to help accentuate the profile include the following:

  Rhinoplasty (nose job)
  Chin augmentation

Just as we discussed the face from top to bottom in previous chapters, we now follow the same pattern here. After a surgical tour of the face, our topics will include such critical issues as recovery times for each procedure; what pain, if any, might be involved; and what to expect before and after surgery.

Treating the Eyes and the Surrounding Area: How the Brow, the Eyes, and the Midface Work in Concert with One Another

One of our patients came in recently and said, "No matter what someone has done, cosmetically speaking, you can always tell their age around the eyes." Although he wasn't entirely accurate, it is true that the delicate and vulnerable skin around the eyes is a little bit like the lines on the cross-section of a tree trunk: look closely enough and you can guess fairly accurately how old someone is.

As we have said repeatedly throughout this book, the best way to deal with the lines around the eyes is to prevent them beforehand: care for your eyes properly so the change never comes. Today's skin-care products—in combination with the appropriate use of Botox and fillers—offer us a huge advantage in this area because they can help to prevent the fine lines associated with the aging process.

Sometimes the eyes are not alone in creating problems for your face; the forehead can be a terrible "upstairs neighbor," drooping and causing the upper lids to look older than they actually are, while sagging and hollow cheeks can act like unruly "downstairs neighbors," adding years to your face.

Does any of this sound familiar so far? It probably does, if you're still reading. The following are the four major issues that we see for surgery when we discuss the eyes:

- **Drooping eyebrows.** Eyebrows that droop can have a tremendous impact on the aging process and can accentuate the laxity of the upper eyelid skin.
- **Upper eyelid laxity.** The skin of the upper eyelid tends to become exaggerated and can start sagging on top of the eyelashes.
- **Lower eyelids.** Problems with your lower eyelids can include puffiness, excess skin, and laxity of the lower eyelid tendons.
- **Midface—cheeks.** As stated earlier, volume loss is one of the main causes of aging in the face, especially around the eyes, the brows, and the cheeks. The shrinkage of tissue here can have a significant impact by creating a flat brow as well as forehead and deep depressions and hollows around the eyes and cheeks. The midface has two main factors that affect it: sagging and volume loss. Both issues should be addressed in midface rejuvenation.

The main thing to remember about the eyes and the surrounding area is that everything affects everything else. For instance, sometimes the cheeks sag and accentuate the bones under the eyelids; at other times, the forehead can weigh down on the upper lids and create more problems. Surgically speaking, how do we treat these problems?

Sagging Brows

Many people come to us with forehead and brow complaints, and for good reason. Your forehead and your brow are often the first to show the signs of aging, and, since your forehead is so exposed, these often dramatic changes become harder and harder to hide.

Your skin loses elasticity; combined with the elements you've endured over time—sun damage, the effects of wind, and gravity's inevitable pull—this results in wrinkles on the forehead, skin that can feel or even look rough, and "frown lines" above and around the brow and the eyes. Your eyebrows may begin to look heavy and to droop.

The illustration below shows how an endoscopic brow lift is done.

Successful brow-lift surgery is a result of good rapport between the patient and the surgeon. For you to develop the necessary rapport with your physician, it helps to know as much as you can about the procedure you're getting before you walk into his or her office. We can provide you with a lot of that information.

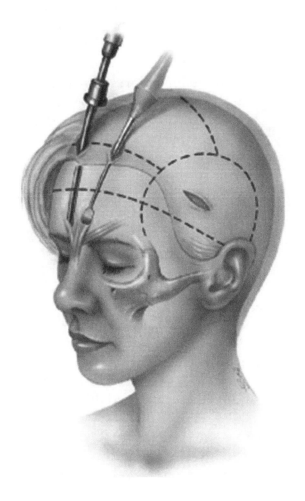

Brow lift

This section will address many of your concerns and provide you with the information you need to begin considering forehead surgery. To try to erase some of the effects of time, heredity, and exposure on your forehead and brow, plastic surgeons focus on two critical aspects of a brow lift:

1. Reducing the activity of overactive muscles
2. Repositioning the eyebrows

By repositioning the eyebrows, your surgeon can greatly reduce the number of wrinkles that exist and relieve some of the effects of drooping that occur at the brow line. By placing the eyebrows in a location that looks more youthful, the surgeon makes the eyes appear more open, and the eyelids will sag less.

It is very important to consider the sex of the patient who is having a forehead lift. Women generally have more arched and higher-positioned eyebrows. The outer part of the brow (tail) should be higher than the inner part. In men, there is generally less of an arch, and the eyebrows should be in a lower position. The tail of the brow is the area that most commonly requires repositioning. The inner portion of the brow near the nose should not be elevated excessively as it will create a "Snoopy" appearance that is not desirable and is a telltale sign of surgery.

For those vertical lines between the brows, which we call the "eleven sign," your doctor might remove part of the *corrugator* muscle that causes them. More recently, we have been advocating caution in doing this. First, the muscles tend to return to action anyway, and second, many nerves run through these muscles, so removing part of them increases the chance of injury. Botox is an excellent alternative to surgery for this area.

Be sure to discuss exactly what your specific needs are during your initial consultation with your physician. Ask what results you can realistically expect, and be clear on how much or how little work you want done. We are seeing amazing results with forehead and brow lifts these days, and there are several reasons for this.

One is that doctors are becoming more experienced at what we consider a more natural change, in which the forehead and brow lifts are not quite as severe as they were in the past. We know that you don't want to have a too tight or surprised look after your lift; you want your forehead to look smoother, your brow and your eyes to droop less, and, above all, your expression to be more youthful and relaxed. These are the ultimate goals of a successful forehead or brow lift.

Many individuals are concerned about scarring after a forehead or brow lift; this is a legitimate concern. However, the forehead and the brow offer numerous places to make incisions, so that scarring can be avoided in the most visible places. Now we can place incisions directly at the hairline or even behind it; by carefully planning and suturing, we leave no visible scarring.

If you are concerned about scarring, discuss the procedure with your doctor and have him or her explain exactly where the incision might be placed. Ask to see "before" and "after" pictures in order to see if the scarring involved is visible; the chances are that you won't be able to tell—even if you are looking for them. In an endoscopic brow lift, we make very small incisions in the scalp along the hairline, and a telescope is used to soften all of the muscles and tissues that bring the eyebrows down. The endoscopic approach is our preferred method for brow lift.

As discussed above, in a three-dimensional brow lift, it's a good idea to leave the inner portion of the eyebrow alone and manipulate the outer portion to create an arch. Balance is the key when performing a successful brow lift. Being excessive or overzealous only gives the patient a surprised "Snoopy" look. We just want to relieve the tension that is bringing the eyebrows down by raising them up a few millimeters.

We don't want people to have a surprised look; if the operation is done right, in a conservative manner, the chances of this are very low. Better still, the length of time before recurrence—of the brows slipping back down—is between five and ten years, so a quality brow lift is fairly long-term.

Occasionally, we recommend having both a brow lift and an eyelid lift (blepharoplasty), or even one of the many face-lift procedures now available, to create an effect of balance and harmony.

When you talk to your doctor, express your concerns about sharpness, contrast, and looking surprised or too tight. Ask which complementary procedures might be available to soften the effects of a forehead or brow lift.

How Does a Forehead or Brow Lift Work, and How Long Does It Take?

We recommend the latest approach in brow and forehead surgery: the endoscopic forehead lift. During this procedure we make several small incisions that are located behind the hairline.

With very advanced endoscopic technology, the incisions must be just less than an inch in size, sometimes as small as half an inch. Then the surgeon can tighten loose skin, remove excess skin, or even remove the muscles that form the "eleven sign" between the eyebrows.

The endoscopic procedure is more delicate and involved than previous forehead and brow-lift procedures were, but, in general, the length of time for surgery is less. The payoff is that the incisions are smaller, the procedure itself is less invasive, and, as a result, the downtime for an endoscopic forehead or brow lift is far less than for other procedures.

Many excellent surgeons still perform coronal, or "open," brow lifts, which require longer incisions. The results of these operations are excellent in the hands of an experienced surgeon. As we have stated repeatedly, discuss your concerns with your surgeon, and if you trust his or her opinion, go ahead with the recommendation.

The endoscopic brow lift procedure will last one to two hours, and typically require general anesthesia, intravenous sedation, or "twilight" anesthesia, in which you are neither fully awake nor fully unconscious.

The Recovery Time and Risks

After a forehead or brow lift, you should expect some bruising and swelling; it can take one to two weeks for this swelling to go down completely. Your physician will remove the sutures in about a week, at which point you will be able to return to work and normal activity. Most physicians will recommend that you avoid strenuous activity for about three weeks.

Throughout this chapter, we discuss the surgical risks associated with various procedures. The reason we are doing so is not to scare you away from surgery but rather to inform you of the potential risks so that you will be more attentive during your consultation and ask your surgeon the right questions. As a general rule, most of the surgical procedures that we discuss have a very low risk of adverse events such as bleeding, infection, scarring, and asymmetry.

With brow lifts, the main risks include facial nerve injury, numbness, and the recurrence of brow drooping. Numbness occurs more frequently with the coronal approach. However, it tends to resolve in a few weeks to a few months and is rarely permanent. The recurrence of drooping tends to occur more frequently with the endoscopic approach and in men.

Eyelid Lift (Blepharoplasty)

In the aging process, the upper eyelids tend to lose volume, become lax, and develop loose skin that hangs down, thereby reducing the beauty of an open eye. The lower eyelids tend to also develop this looseness; however, the supporting structures tend to weaken, which causes puffiness of the lower eyes due to the protrusion of the internal fat pads. In addition, the area under the eyes (adjacent to the cheeks) tends to become more and more hollow as we age, which results in skeletonization around the eyes.

Blepharoplasty, or eyelid-lift surgery, has undergone a significant transformation in the past decade. In the past, blepharoplasty routinely involved the removal of significant fat, skin, and muscle from the eyelid and brow areas in order to obtain "youthful" eyes.

Unfortunately, this approach often resulted in a trend toward hollowness of the eye area and a significant "catlike" look of the corner of the eyes, which was unnatural and changed the entire appearance of the patient. Complications were also more common with this type of procedure.

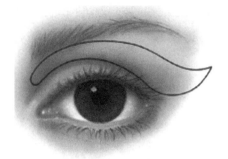

Upper blepharoplasty incision

Today we know that the aging changes around the eyes do not simply involve sagging skin. There are multiple components to consider before performing any eyelid lift surgery, such as hollowness, loss of skin elasticity, drooping of the eyebrows and cheek fat pads, and weakness of the supporting eyelid structures (which leads to puffiness under the eyes).

We certainly don't want to address just the eyes without considering the rest of the face, so when we evaluate aging eyes, we also want to consider how the forehead and the midface-cheek area will affect the eyes and be affected in return.

The figures on this page show the location of the blepharoplasty incision and what facial plastic surgeons consider to be the ideal brow position. The inner aspect of the brow should be in the same plane as the outer aspect of the nose and nostrils. The tail or outer aspect of the brow should follow a line drawn from the nose to the outer portion of the eyelids. The inner portion of the brow is typically fuller. In women, there is usually a soft arch on the outer aspect of the eyebrow. In men, the eyebrows should be positioned lower and should not have an exaggerated arch.

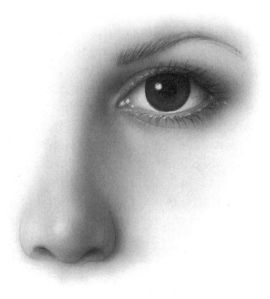

The "ideal" eyebrow position

Through a better understanding of eyelid anatomy, facial analysis, and aging changes, today's sophisticated plastic surgeons often utilize a very different approach to blepharoplasty. Depending on your physician's skill and expertise, the approach can include the use of fillers or injectables (such as Restylane, Juvéderm, and Botox), fractionated laser skin resurfacing, conservative surgical eyelid lift (blepharoplasty), multilevel fat grafting (MFG), endoscopic brow lift, and/or midface-lift to create the most natural-looking and long-lasting results.

Below are "before" and "after" pictures of a successful blepharoplasty.

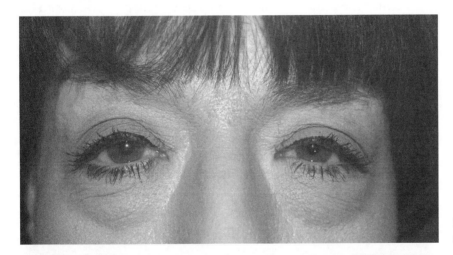

Before blepharoplasty and MFG

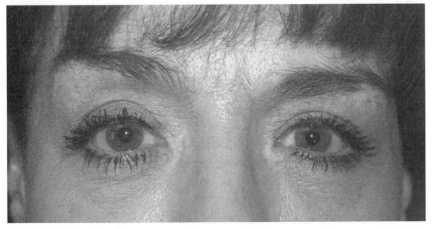

After blepharoplasty and MFG

By carefully examining the eyes in relation to the rest of the face, and considering multiple complementary procedures to create a full and youthful expression, the surgeon gives each individual a personalized approach to his or her eyelid lift. The results are natural and involve minimal risks, complications, or downtime.

How Does Blepharoplasty Work and How Long Does It Take?

Blepharoplasty is eyelid surgery in which excess skin—sometimes in combination with fat and muscle—is contoured from either the upper or the lower eyelids. The procedure can be performed simultaneously on the upper and the lower eyelids.

Your facial plastic surgeon will make tiny incisions in the creases of skin (this cuts down on scarring and makes the incisions barely noticeable). For upper-lid blepharoplasty, your physician will make the incision in the crease of the eyelid. For lower-lid blepharoplasty, your plastic surgeon will make the incision on the inner part of the eyelid, thereby avoiding an outside scar (the *transconjunctival* approach). In some people, it is necessary to also make an incision just below the lashes.

Once the incision is made, your physician will separate the skin from the muscle and the fatty tissue that lie underneath. Once that part of the procedure is performed, the surgeon will

WHAT YOUR DOCTOR DOESN'T KNOW COULD HURT YOU!

If you are considering an eyelid lift (*blepharoplasty*), make sure that your doctor knows if you have dry eyes, stinging eyes, or issues with your cornea; if you do have any of these conditions, you might not be an appropriate candidate for upper blepharoplasty. In fact, we recommend that most people be evaluated by an ophthalmologist before they have this or any other surgical procedure around the eyes.

remove or reposition a specific amount of excess fat before contouring the muscle and trimming the sagging skin for the desired effect. The incision will then be closed with fine sutures.

An upper or lower blepharoplasty is performed on an outpatient basis. Your plastic surgeon will use a local anesthetic—along with sedation—to relax you during the surgical procedure. The surgery will take anywhere from one to two hours, depending on how many—and which—lids are being done. Complementary procedures such as endoscopic browlift, midface lift, and/or multilevel fat grafting may be performed at the same time.

The Recovery Time and Risks

You should give yourself a full week to completely recover. Although most people can return to work in several days, vigorous activity should be avoided for the first week. Bruising and swelling take about seven to ten days to clear up enough for people to feel comfortable in social gatherings.

In the hands of an experienced surgeon, blepharoplasty is safe with predictable results. The main issues that you need to be aware of occur with lower-lid blepharoplasty. The lower lids are very finicky. Aggressive surgical intervention after an inappropriate preoperative evaluation can lead to unwanted changes in the lid's shape and position, lowering the lid and leading to a rounding and a widening of the eyes (*lower lid malposition*). This can lead to an excess showing of the white portion of the eye (*scleral show*) and an outward turning of the lower lid (*ectropion*). Other risks of blepharoplasty include bleeding, asymmetry, persistent eyelid hooding, injury to the internal muscles, and dry eyes.

Through a better understanding of eyelid anatomy, facial analysis, and aging changes, today's modern plastic surgeons often utilize a very different approach to blepharoplasty.

Midface Rejuvenation

To rejuvenate the midface region, which is the area from the lower eyelids to above the upper lip, careful consideration must be paid to how this region interacts with and affects the eyelids.

In the past, a face-lift was a face-lift was a face-lift; one procedure covered all, from the forehead to the eyes to the cheeks to the chin, producing uneven and unnatural-looking results for entire generations of plastic-surgery seekers. Today, many surgeons specialize in what is known as a *midface-lift*, in which the region between the eyelids and above the lips is specifically addressed.

People who seek a midface-lift are typically concerned with issues like trying to soften and reduce deep "laugh lines" (nasolabial folds). They also want to restore luster and fullness to their cheeks, which can hollow and sharpen over time. The three-dimensional midface-lift can address all of these issues and more, if you also discuss with your doctor complementary procedures (such as MFG and fillers) to reduce the roughness and wrinkling of aging skin.

Midface implants can also be extremely useful in rejuvenating the midface by restoring volume loss and providing three-dimensional lift. Traditional cheek implants have unfortunately given midface implants a bad name because they were placed in the wrong anatomic position – high up in the cheek bone. This exaggerated look was a telltale sign of bad plastic surgery for much of the 1980s and 1990s. With today's techniques, popularized by Dr. William Binder, midface implants are placed into a more normal anatomic position, resulting in a natural, aesthetic outcome.

How Does a Midface-Lift Work and How Long Does It Take?

Technological advance of the endoscope allows surgeons to reduce deep "laugh lines" and increase fullness in the midface with minimal invasiveness, using specialized tools. When your procedure is performed with an endoscope, the incisions will be smaller and can be camouflaged by natural facial features, such as the hairline or the front of the ear. The tissue is fixed in the desired position by sutures or ENDOTINE midface fixation system. The ENDOTINE midface fixation is a novel system that allows mechanical fixation throughout the postoperative healing period and eventually resorbs as scar tissue takes over. This system can also be utilized in fixating brow lifts.

Depending on the severity of the problem and your desired outcome, an endoscopic midface-lift can take from one to two hours to perform. It is an outpatient procedure.

The Recovery Time and Risks

The endoscope improves precision. Because we can reach and manipulate the muscle and fat deposits throughout the face, we can sculpt the features more precisely, preserving your natural facial contours and creating a more natural-looking, vibrant effect.

Because of the type of surgical manipulation that is done in the cheek area, the recuperation from an endoscopic midface-lift tends to be a bit longer than for blepharoplasty and endoscopic forehead lifts. Patients will generally have swelling for about two to three weeks.

The risks of a midface-lift are very similar to those of a brow lift. The main issues that can arise are injury of the facial nerves, numbness of the cheeks, and infection. The recovery time for this procedure tends to be a bit longer than for other facial rejuvenation operations.

Rejuvenating the Lower Face and the Neck Together

It would be easy to say that a face is a face is a face and treat the sum of the parts as if they were the whole, but as we can clearly see, the eyes contain very specific problems that require very specific procedures. The wide expanse of the brow, for instance, requires one type of product or procedure, whereas the intricate, delicate, and extremely sensitive skin around the eyes requires another skill set entirely.

Not only must we consider how to treat each part of the face separately, we must also consider how they work together. Your

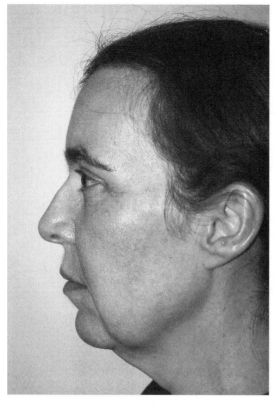

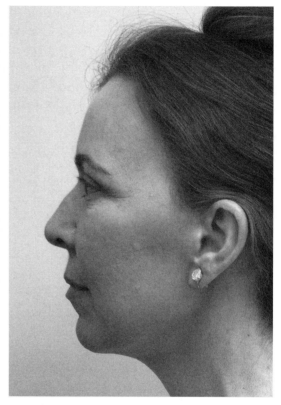

Before face and neck lift

After face and neck lift

surgeon will often recommend two procedures to increase the effectiveness of one—or even both.

Likewise, the lower face and the neck have unique features that require separate but equal attention.

The Lower Face

We have seen how forehead and brow lifts can address trouble areas such as deep furrows between the eyebrows, wrinkles on the forehead, and drooping brows. In addition, we have learned that both MFG and midface-lifts address deep "laugh lines" and hollow cheeks.

Now we turn our attention to issues concerning the lower face, which is considered to be the jawline and the underside of the chin. The lower face can greatly benefit from such complementary procedures as MFG, chin implants, fillers, and laser resurfacing.

Currently, there are several face-lift techniques that can successfully address the lower face. We will divide them into the following categories:

- Skin-only, subcutaneous face-lifts
- Superficial musculo-aponeurotic system (SMAS) face-lifts
- Deep-plane face-lifts

WHAT IS A MINI-FACE-LIFT?

We wish to exert a word of caution here about mini-face-lift procedures. Every "mini" lift is different, depending on the surgeon who is performing the procedure, so please don't ask your surgeon for a "mini" lift! Most "mini" lifts are less involved than legitimate face-lifts (such as limited incision and/or limited dissection), whereas others are nothing but sham surgery being performed by unqualified physicians.

In other words, most legitimate mini-face-lifts are still *major* surgical procedures, so don't be fooled by the name. You should ask your doctor why he or she calls the procedure a "mini" procedure. You also should make sure that your doctor is actually a qualified surgeon—that is, certified by the American Board of Facial Plastic and Reconstructive Surgery, the American Board of Plastic Surgery, or the American Board of Otolaryngology (with sub-specialty training in facial plastic surgery).

Many unqualified surgeons and physicians perform mini-face-lifts in their offices under local anesthesia because they don't have the credentials to perform them at the hospitals or the ambulatory surgical centers at which they otherwise work. Once again, knowledge is power; knowing the right questions to ask before a consultation can greatly reduce your risk of problems with such procedures later.

How Does a Lower-Face Face-Lift
Work and How Long Does It Take?

The superficial musculo-aponeurotic system (SMAS) is a layer of tissue just below the skin that serves as the foundation and structural support for the lower face. Subcutaneous face-lifts essentially elevate the skin without touching the SMAS. For the most part, SMAS face-lifts use this layer to fortify the face-lift. Deep-plane face-lifts penetrate the SMAS to lift the lax tissue.

Most sophisticated facial plastic surgeons employ either the SMAS or the deep-plane face-lift. Many surgeons have excellent success with subcutaneous face-lifts as well. Our recommendation is to make sure that your surgeon has a long track record with the technique that is to be utilized. Experience and expertise are key.

CORPORATE MEDICINE AND THE FACE-LIFT

There is currently a multitude of "face-lift clinics" that woo unsuspecting individuals with exaggerated promises of life-changing procedures at extremely low prices. At these places, "consultants" who are not physicians evaluate the people. These individuals are rewarded by the parent corporations for the number of surgeries they schedule. For the most part, they have no medical background to enable them to screen for life-threatening medical conditions or contraindications to surgery.

In these "clinics," physicians see patients only after the services have been paid for, and they rarely follow up after the immediate postoperative period. These are exactly the type of settings that should be avoided, because they have a big potential for major medical errors. We really believe that plastic surgery should be performed with the highest level of ethics and medical care, with appropriate physician evaluation and follow-up.

You need to look carefully at your surgeon's "before" and "after" photos to make sure that his or her aesthetic eye matches yours. This is the most crucial aspect of facial rejuvenation surgery. Some surgeons love the overpulled look, whereas others prefer a more natural look. Finally, make sure that your doctor performs facial rejuvenation procedures on a routine basis. You don't want a "breast expert" performing you face-lift procedure.

Lower face-lifts are outpatient procedures that take about two to three hours.

The Recovery Time and Risks

The recovery time for face-lift procedures on the lower face will depend on the technique employed by your doctor. Most people will be able to return to routine activity in about eight to ten days. Exercise can be resumed in three weeks.

The main risks of face-lifts on the lower face include bleeding, poor blood flow to the skin, scarring, numbness, and injury of the facial nerves. Overall, the biggest problem is that 2 to 5 percent of individuals will have some blood collection under the skin in the first two to three days after surgery. Most of these hematomas, as they are called, will be limited and can be taken care of in the office.

Occasionally, however, hematomas have to be urgently cleared up in the operating room. Men have a higher chance than women of developing hematomas. Smokers also tend to have a higher risk, due to bad circulation, which can lead to scarring and loss of tissue. Most face-lift surgeons do not operate on smokers for this reason, unless they stop smoking two weeks before and two weeks after surgery. (Nicotine gum and patches must also be avoided.)

The Neck

For many people, the neck is where some of the most obvious signs of aging first appear. Like the forehead, the neck is extremely visible and hard to camouflage; it is also particularly sensitive and, as such, quite vulnerable to the effects of the elements and aging. Over time, the skin of the neck has a tendency to become loose and slack; deposits of fat and flaps of tissue can make you appear older than your actual age.

Some of the factors that contribute to the aesthetic problems that develop around the neck include the following:

- **Loosening muscles.** In the neck area, the SMAS converges to form the platysma muscle on each side of the neck. These muscles begin to lose their structure and elasticity and this can contribute to loose skin and the wattles that affect so many of us as we age. Unfortunately, there are no exercises that can make the neck of the skin firmer.
- **Fat—it's not just at your waistline anymore.** As we age, deposits of excess fat can accumulate in the neck and under the chin to create an undesirable effect.
- **Beneath the skin—and beyond.** Like the rest of your face, your neck has various layers that work together as well as independently. Just as your forehead can be a bad "upstairs neighbor" to your eye region, so too can the submuscular area of the neck weaken the foundation of your appearance. In this case, the underlying structure of the neck begins to suffer from the sagging of loose excess skin and muscle in the area.
- **Loss of skin elasticity.** The skin of the neck is particularly susceptible to a loss of elasticity with age, and even as it sags, it continues to lose the sense of fullness that we equate with youth.

The neck is one of the only areas that is not amenable to non-invasive rejuvenation. Fortunately, having a neck lift can address each of these issues. In some cases, a neck lift is absolutely the only solution to restore and revitalize your appearance. In most cases, face-lifts and neck lifts are performed simultaneously, thereby creating a more natural-looking appearance.

During the procedure, your physician will do the following as necessary:

- Join and tighten the muscles of the neck, creating a firmer muscle base

- Remove excess fat deposits
- Trim excess skin and smooth the skin for a taut, more youthful neckline

How Does a Neck Lift Work and How Long Does It Take?

Speak with your doctor openly and honestly about your expectations of a neck lift. Your goals will customize the procedure you get. Depending on your specific needs and goals, a customized neck lift will consist of the following procedures:

- **Skin and platysma lift.** The skin lift consists of lifting and tightening the skin in combination with the platysma muscles along the neck. By removing excess skin, the surgeon can create a more youthful facial appearance. The incisions for an isolated neck lift can be placed behind the ears, thereby avoiding any visible scars.
- **Platysmaplasty.** A platysmaplasty is a procedure in which the underlying muscles are tightened and the fat is removed. This procedure provides more dramatic results for individuals whose underlying neck tissue is very lax. The incision tends to be just beneath the chin in a hidden crease. Many people also undergo simultaneous liposuction of excess fat deposits through this tiny incision.
- **Liposuction.** Many people will develop some fatty deposits under the neck during the aging process. This is an excellent area for conservative liposuction during a neck lift. Younger individuals may even be candidates for neck liposuction as a stand-alone procedure to rejuvenate the neck area.

A neck lift is an outpatient cosmetic procedure and typically takes from two to three hours.

The Recovery Time and Risks

The recovery time for a neck lift is relatively short, and most people can return to work and recreational activities in about one week.

The risks of a neck lift are very similar to those of a face-lift.

In addition, aggressive liposuction in this region can sometimes lead to "cobra" neck deformity. This occurs when the neck muscles are not addressed at the same time, and this can cause excess visibility of the banding.

The Profile: Surgery on the Nose and the Chin

Although the nose is technically part of the midface and the chin can rightfully be considered part of the lower face, for our purposes we combine them in a separate category to achieve a profile that is balanced in both perspective and fullness.

The profile is certainly important enough to be considered a separate entity, for even though we see only our full face staring straight ahead when we look in a mirror, others just as often see our profiles coming or going.

Likewise, the nose and the chin often work together to give balance to the face, both in full frontal view and when viewed from the side. For this reason, we thought they should have "separate but equal" treatment.

The Nose

We can't underestimate the importance of the nose in terms of the overall aesthetics of the face. When we are trying to create a balanced, symmetrical appearance, the nose is literally the center of the face, and everything else radiates from that center. It is therefore very important that you consider your nose when you are consulting about the rest of your face.

Although the nose at first seems impenetrable to age—it doesn't get wrinkles like the forehead or wattles like the neck— the nose is not, in fact, entirely immune to the effects of aging. With each passing decade, the nose can start to look longer and can even droop. The nasal skin changes dramatically with age; it tends to become either thicker or thinner.

Most people think that a nose job, or rhinoplasty, is only for those who consider their nose too big, too long, too wide, too flat, or otherwise somehow too unsightly. These are indeed the most common reasons for seeking a nose job. However, as goes the nose, so goes the rest of the face; by creating a more youthful-looking nose, we can create a more youthful appearance on the rest of the face as well. In other words, one should not overlook the nose when one is trying to reverse the signs of aging.

While reviewing your desired results for a nose job and the alternatives that are currently available, your physician will discuss various issues with you, such as the size, shape, and texture of your desired nose as well as its functionality. You will certainly want to know if your new nose will affect your breathing and your sinuses, for example.

We've all seen noses that look like they've been done, and we want to avoid that at all costs. As with every other aspect of your face, we want your nose to look natural, balanced, and symmetrical in relation to the rest of your features, such as the lips and the chin, which can have a significant impact on the perception of the nose.

How Does Rhinoplasty Work and How Long Does It Take?

Rhinoplasty is one of the most common yet challenging cosmetic procedures. The key to a successful outcome resides in creating a natural-looking, well-proportioned nose without sacrificing an individual's breathing function. Your desires, ethnicity, and facial proportions are of the utmost importance in determining the proper rhinoplasty procedure. Ask your doctor if digital morphing systems can help you to see the future changes.

A systematic approach is utilized for the treatment plan, which is almost always unique to each individual. The following components are evaluated and addressed:

- Age
- Ethnicity
- Skin thickness
- Nasal profile
- Frontal aesthetics of the nose

- Tip and base of the nose
- Nasal-lip relationship
- Nasal-chin relationship
- History of trauma
- Breathing system: septum, nasal valves, cartilage, allergies, and sinus disease

OPEN VERSUS CLOSED RHINOPLASTY

Once you start researching nose jobs, you will hear a lot about whether your surgeon does "open" or "closed" rhinoplasty. An open rhinoplasty (also referred to as the external approach) uses a small incision under the nose to allow direct visibility of the tip. Conversely, the closed, or endonasal, approach utilizes only internal incisions to access the nasal anatomy.

Both approaches are excellent, and the outcome again depends on the expertise of your surgeon. There has been a recent trend toward performing open rhinoplasty for more complicated primary and revisional rhinoplasty procedures.

Discuss the matter with your surgeon. Do not count out a surgeon who performs an open rhinoplasty procedure because you have heard that the scarring and/or healing is worse. Most sophisticated plastic surgeons will be able to perform both types of procedures and will recommend what they think will be best for your particular nose.

Proceed with Caution

Rhinoplasty is often considered the most challenging plastic-surgical procedure. Thus, you have to be even more certain of your surgeon's qualifications and experience. Your surgeon should be certified by the American Board of Facial Plastic and Reconstructive Surgery, the American Board of Otolaryngology, or the American Board of Plastic Surgery. He or she should perform at least thirty to forty operations per year. As always, you should review "before" and "after" photos to make sure that you see eye to eye with your doctor. If you are having a bump removed, digital imaging can help you to visualize the final outcome. Changes in the tip, however, are less dramatic in digital imaging.

A rhinoplasty begins with the plastic surgeon making incisions inside the nasal cavity. After that, the cartilage and bone of the nose are sculpted, shaped, or in some cases even reconstructed to the desired specifications of the preoperative treatment plan. The skin from the nose is then sutured carefully, and bandages are applied to prevent infection and promote proper healing.

Rhinoplasty is usually an outpatient procedure; it can take from one to four hours, depending on the severity of the procedure. In most people, you will see no exterior, noticeable scars.

The Recovery Time and Risks

The recovery time for rhinoplasty is generally one to two weeks. Initially you will have a splint on your nose, but it will be removed one week later. Some individuals will have nasal packing, a small tampon that will prevent bleeding. Immediately after the surgery, you will be seen by your physician several times in the first ten days. After that you will typically be seen every three months for one year, then annually after that. Follow-up is a critical component of rhinoplasty, because the nose will continue to heal in the first twelve months. Make sure that your surgeon carefully follows his or her patients for a long time after surgery.

The nose heals in a completely different way from the rest of the face. The swelling tends to take several months to settle down. This swelling will have a tremendous impact on your appearance, so you have to be patient until it is all gone.

The chances of having a bad outcome from rhinoplasty are directly related to the experience of your surgeon and the degree of complexity of the surgery. Your expectations must be in line with what the surgeon can deliver in results. Preoperative communication is so important to avoid misunderstandings. There are two types of issues that can arise from rhinoplasty:

- **Immediate postoperative.** In the immediate postoperative period, rhinoplasty has an extremely safe track record. However, the standard risks are bleeding, infection, scarring, skin breakout, and headaches.
- **Long-term.** The long-term complications are much more problematic. The nose heals very differently from almost

any other body part. In fact, the nose tends to evolve for years after surgery. If the basic principles of the procedure are not considered at the time of surgery, major adverse events can occur. These problems can include asymmetry, collapse of the nasal valves, nasal breathing issues, scarring, and poor aesthetic outcome. As a result, revision rhinoplasty has become a big business, because there is a high percentage of people who experience long-term issues.

This section is not meant to scare you from having your nose done; it is simply meant to make sure that you pick your surgeon carefully. In the hands of the right surgeon, the results can be very positive.

The Chin

Facial appearances can be deceiving. Particularly in terms of the relationship between the nose and the chin, what others see is not always what you actually have, and the latter relationship is occasionally ignored by some physicians. For instance, most individuals with an undersized chin are not aware that this feature results in the illusion of a larger nose.

This is another example of the importance of making sure that whatever procedure you have done is thoroughly examined beforehand to determine how it will affect the rest of your face. Without a thorough consultation before the surgery, you may be surprised that changing your nose, for instance, changes your chin—even though all you had was a nose job.

What happens when you are dissatisfied with your chin, in general, and you haven't had any other procedures done? Many people come to us complaining about the size, shape, and/or texture of their chins. Fortunately, there are many options for chin augmentation these days. The most common approach is to use a chin implant to achieve the desired shape and size. Fillers such as Radiesse and/or laser resurfacing can be used as complementary procedures to address roughness or other texture issues.

Facial implants can be an excellent option for people who are unhappy with their facial structure and who want to achieve a desired effect by modifying the lower face, in general, and the chin, in particular. Chin implants are an effective way to change the appearance of a weak chin by strengthening the profile and giving better proportion to the face. They are also commonly used as a complementary procedure to lower face-lifts to enhance the jawline in individuals who have had jaw bone decay.

These days, chin implants are formed from a safe, solid silicone material. Thanks to modern technology and a skilled plastic surgeon, a silicone chin implant will look and feel just like the real thing. We want you to feel as good as you look, so we work hard to create a natural-looking, balanced effect with all our chin implants.

How Does a Chin Implant Work and How Long Does It Take?

During the initial consultation, your surgeon should carefully evaluate your dentition to make sure that you don't have any major bite deformities that actually require orthognathic (jaw) surgery. Once the appropriate evaluation has been done, you and your plastic surgeon will select the correct size and shape of the implant before the procedure. A chin implant is usually performed under general anesthesia.

During the procedure, the surgeon will make a small incision along the inside of your lower lip or under the chin. Due to their size and placement, these incisions will leave no visible scarring. The doctor will then gently insert the implant through this incision, adjusting as necessary for optimum results.

A chin implant is a relatively short procedure. It takes half an hour to an hour, depending on the size of the implant.

The Recovery Time and Risks

Recovery time for a chin implant is fairly minimal; most people need five to ten days to fully recover. The swelling may take a bit longer to recede. The final results are evident at three months.

RECOVERY TIMES BY PROCEDURE

How long will the recovery from your plastic surgery take? Recovery times differ by patient, but the following average times can give you a general idea when you are planning for any of the following procedures:

- **Forehead or brow lift.** For most people, the recovery time will not exceed two weeks, but individuals may still be advised to avoid strenuous activities for longer periods.
- **Blepharoplasty.** Bruising and swelling takes about seven to ten days to clear up enough for people to feel comfortable in social gatherings.
- **Endoscopic midface lift.** Since the incisions for the endoscope tend to be much smaller and the invasion less severe, recovery can take less than a week. The swelling with a midface lift will last about three to four weeks.
- **Face-lift or neck lift.** The recovery time for either a face-lift or a neck lift is relatively short; most people return to work and recreational activities in about seven to ten days.
- **Chin or cheek implant.** Recovery time for either procedure is minimal; most people need only seven to ten days to fully recover.
- **Rhinoplasty.** The recovery time is generally one to two weeks.
- **Neck liposuction.** Normal activities can be undertaken in two to four days, and return to normal activities is possible in less than a week.

Chin implants are extremely safe, with excellent track records. As with all procedures, careful considerations can minimize bad outcomes. Even in the hands of the most adept surgeon, however, there are some potential risks. These are bleeding, infection that requires the removal of the implant, poor positioning or displacement of the implant, poor aesthetics, and nerve injury that results in numbness of the lower lip. These complications occur in 1 to 2 percent of the cases.

Questions, Answers, and Preparations: What to Expect Before Surgery

Plastic surgery has made significant advances over the past two decades. The figures below are before and after photos of Mary Jo Buttafuoco, who developed facial paralysis and asymmetry from a gunshot wound to the head region. She underwent a customized face-lift procedure, blepharoplasty, MFG, Radiesse, and Botox treatments. The operation, which was performed by Dr. Azizzadeh, was featured on *The Oprah Winfrey Show*.

Now you've seen the considerable variety of cosmetic surgeries on the market today. If you have also committed to having some surgery, your next step is to begin to make plans for the procedure itself. First, however, you must be fully prepared.

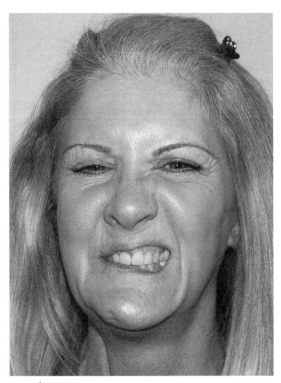

Mary Jo Buttafuoco, preop

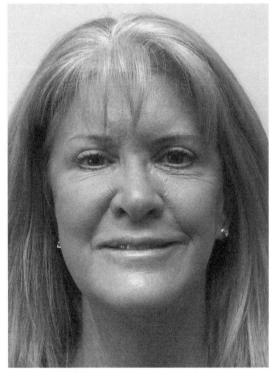

Mary Jo Buttafuoco, postop

There are many steps on the way to a plastic surgeon's office. The most important steps you'll ever take before you have facial plastic surgery are the following:

- **Ask questions.** It is very important that you feel comfortable speaking with your plastic surgeon; if you don't, he or she may not be right for you. His or her expertise lies in the surgical procedure you are paying to have performed, but just as important is the doctor's skill in making you feel comfortable about the procedure. Information is as important as anesthesia or antibacterial soap when you have plastic surgery, and questions are the ultimate tool for obtaining that information.

- **Get answers.** Of course, questions are useless without answers—so get those, too. Don't be satisfied with just any answers to your questions; get the right answers for *your* questions. Doctors can easily slip into a pattern of assuming that their patients understand complicated principles and foreign concepts when, in fact, the patients are simply too intimidated or insecure to say that they don't. If you do understand something, that's wonderful; if not, ask until you do.

- **Prepare thoroughly.** Before surgery, your physician will give you plenty of lists and handouts to follow so that you can be prepared for the procedure. These include checklists of what not to do before surgery—such as eat or take aspirin—as well as various safety protocols you must follow in the weeks, days, and hours before the procedure. Follow these steps precisely and make sure that you are fully prepared before the surgery. We have seen many people who don't take these instructions seriously. After reading this book, you should not be one of them!

Aftercare, Pain, and Downtime: What to Expect after Surgery

As we have discussed, some of these surgeries are noninvasive, whereas others require considerable downtime. How will you know which is which? This book describes general recovery times and the sort of pain our patients feel, but your doctor will be better able to discuss such specifics with you on a case-by-case basis.

The best way to avoid being surprised after surgery is to be prepared before surgery. This depends foremost on choosing the right doctor. The basis for this choice is not just how attentive the physician is before surgery but also how attentive he or she will be after surgery. You should inquire about this ahead of time.

It's easy to focus on the issues you must deal with before the procedure and neglect the issues that will come up after, but we

DISCUSSING RISK IS THE BEST WAY TO AVOID IT

Every surgery contains some risk, no matter how major or minor it might appear. Complications arise, mistakes can be made, genetic conditions can materialize, and a host of other variables can come into play to increase the risk of any surgery. The best way to avoid risk is not only to prepare for it but also to discuss it thoroughly with your doctor beforehand.

Discuss with your doctor such things as the following:

- Whether you smoke
- If you are pregnant or have other medical conditions
- What medications you are taking

This preliminary discussion makes your primary physician aware of any and all potential risks involved in your upcoming surgery—and helps both of you to avoid them.

are stressing that you should be equally concerned with both phases of your surgery. In short, ask, ask, and ask! Ask who will be tending to your care directly after the surgery. Ask how often you'll see the doctor in the recovery room. Ask how long the recovery will take, where it will take place, who will be your point person, and when and how many follow-up visits should be scheduled.

If your doctor is not seeing you after surgery, that's not the right doctor for you. A physician's assistant or a nurse should *not* be the primary consultant after surgery or, for that matter, during regular periodic follow-ups. The consultation should not be done by anyone other than the primary physician.

Most of all, be patient about your recovery time; it's taken fifty years to age, so you've got to give your surgery time to heal. When you know ahead of time how long it's supposed to take to heal, you can avoid the panic of unrealistic postsurgical expectations.

One thing we especially urge is that if you have questions, go see your doctor before you pick up the phone to ask your friends. In many cases, friends just make it worse; they seem to support your anxiety during this already vulnerable time. In our experience, it's not really helpful to have your friends fill your head with too many stories of how their recovery "didn't take nearly as long," how "it's not supposed to look like that," or "when Sylvia had her face-lift, she was playing tennis by Tuesday."

The support you receive from the medical staff at your physician's office is extremely important. We repeat, this is something to observe before surgery, not after; if the staff isn't responding well before surgery, they're going to do the same thing after surgery. If that's the case, then that particular doctor is not right for you.

Choosing a doctor is a critical step in seeking the help you deserve; take it seriously, and don't be so afraid of or intimidated by your doctor that you feel locked into a decision once you've made it. If your doctor is not performing his or her presurgical duties to your standards, consider getting another doctor entirely. This isn't just your right, it's your responsibility.

The next chapters will help you to choose the right doctor for you and will also answer any additional questions you may have before deciding to have surgery. You should be reading this book *before* you've committed to major facial surgery; if this is not the case, discuss with your doctor how to reschedule so you can be better prepared. The best way to avoid being surprised after surgery is to be prepared before surgery.

9

Beverly Hills Celebrity Beauty Secrets

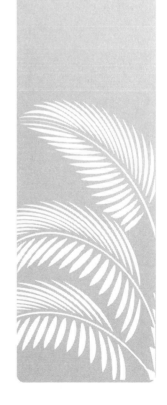

> If you stay in Beverly Hills too long, you become a Mercedes.
>
> —ROBERT REDFORD

Y ou've heard of the South Beach diet, the Laguna Beach diet, the Mediterranean diet, and even the Beverly Hills diet. Then there's *6 Weeks to a Hollywood Body*, *The 30-Minute Celebrity Makeover Miracle*, *The A-List Workout*, *The Ultimate New York Body Plan*, and *The Hollywood Trainer Weight-Loss Plan*.

There is a plethora of diet books from the rich, the famous, and the powerful and a slew of exercise books from celebrities, the A-list, and the beautiful. To this list we now add a book to revitalize and rejuvenate your face by two Beverly Hills experts. This is the book that shares insider tips about celebrity skin-care secrets and tantalizing tidbits about the habits of the beautiful, the youthful, and the fabulous.

The Top Five Secrets the Celebrities Don't Want You to Know

Do you want to know a secret? Do you want to know what celebrities don't want you to know? Celebrities *hate* high-definition television (HD-TV). It's too much like reality: it shows off every flaw, every line, every wrinkle, every sag, every blemish, and every bit of discoloration. Think about that the next time you watch those A-listers strolling down the red carpet on your flat-screen HD-TV.

Celebrities are in the business of being beautiful. Furthermore, they hate aging. Hollywood is a young town—maybe not in actual years, but in spirit. Youth is coveted and age is barely tolerated. Although there are notable exceptions of the Oscar-winning performance by a fiftysomething or sixtysomething actor or actress, it's the young ones who are drawing in moviegoers at the box office and pulling huge Nielsen ratings on TV.

To compete, celebrities start young to work at staying young. They begin early, not only preventing skin damage but also correcting "flaws" and maintaining "perfection" through products and procedures both periodic and routine. The most extreme take drastic measures with unflattering results. The moderates take a long-term approach, doing things subtly, slowly, and regularly to achieve results that are natural, flattering and—in the best cases—flawless.

Even those who claim to have never had a procedure done—well, you and I can both tell when a celebrity has been a lifelong member of the Youthful Face and Features Club, which only proves that prevention, maintenance, and lifelong skin care can work wonders.

In the day-to-day reality of a celebrity's life, the quest is to look and feel more youthful, radiant, and glamorous. Does this sound familiar? That's precisely the point: celebrities want the same things that you and I do; it's just that they actually know how to go about getting it. Fortunately, so do we.

Here are our top five celebrity beauty secrets:

1. **They are no different from you.** We always like to say, "Celebrities wash their faces one pore at a time, just as you do." They really do. They have to go outside and expose themselves to harsh winds, bright sunlight, and air pollution, just as you do. They get up early, go to work, come home and eat something, and stay up late, just as you do. They have the same insecurities and fears that you have.

2. **They do a few things differently from you.** Unlike you, however, celebrities see beauty and youthfulness as an investment in their future. They do not troubleshoot when things go awry; instead, they are always diligently on the lookout for what to do *before* things go awry. You could call them "vigilant about perfection," always researching the latest development in lotions, potions, products, and procedures. We have certainly been charged with keeping up with our celebrity clients, just in the sheer volume of information they bring to each consultation.

3. **They think nothing of getting the latest procedure done.** Many of you consider the products and procedures outlined in this book as big deals or huge undertakings. Not celebrities—they literally use lasers and skin care like the average person uses a toothbrush and goes for a dental cleaning. They know all the details and can quote both recovery times and risks to us verbatim. Most of all, they know the results.

4. **They are fearless about looking flawless.** You would think that people who make a living from their looks would be *more* cautious about having procedures done—but just the opposite is true. That's because celebrities do their homework, find the best physician available, and budget accordingly for having the right work done at the right time by the best person for the job. When you factor in those three critical variables, the risk goes down and the rewards go up.

5. **They know that beauty is an endless quest.** Just as the rest of us plan on working well into retirement, celebrities never give up on looking youthful, glamorous, and flawless. You might say they have two jobs: the first is what made them celebrities in the first place (acting, singing, sports, politics), and the second is what keeps them celebrities year after year (looking youthful, glamorous, and flawless).

Celebrities want the same things that you and I do, it's just that they actually know how to go about getting it.

Famous Places, Famous Faces

It seems that every famous place thinks it has the right to tell you how to lose weight and tone up. There are few places in the world as renowned for beauty, glitz, and glamour as Beverly Hills.

You can point to the exclusive police force, the luxury hotels, the million-dollar starter homes, the swanky shops, and the purses filled with pooches as the exterior signs of our inherent sense of lavishness, luxury, and a lush life.

People come from all over the world to visit our hundreds of spas, dermatologists, plastic surgeons, and recovery centers. Every day we treat people from all over the world. Here we have specialists who do things that no one else does—and that no one ever dreamed possible before—for individuals who demand the latest, greatest products and procedures from all over the world. If there is a new product on the market, our celebrity clients don't just want it; they demand it. If there is a new procedure on the market, we don't just look into it; we tend to specialize in it.

The Beverly Hills Beauty Program

The Beverly Hills Beauty Program is a proactive, generational regimen that combines preventive maintenance (in your twenties and thirties), various surgical and nonsurgical rejuvenating procedures (in your forties), and a combination of restorative procedures and maintenance regimens (in your fifties and beyond). This program is based on our experience with our celebrity clients. It provides a long-term plan to help you care for, preserve, and rejuvenate your face. You can start it anytime you like; it's never too late or too early.

This is the approach we often use on our most conscientious and famous clients. Of course, we can't tell you their names, but they have been the inspiration in developing a long-term plan in preventing the aging process, maintaining a youthful appearance, and rejuvenating the face.

A Program for the Ages—to Make You Feel Ageless

The Beverly Hills Beauty Program is built on three principles that provide a solid foundation on which to construct your facial rejuvenation experience. These include the following:

1. **Prevention.** The first part of the program you can actually do yourself. That's because much of what we work so diligently to repair in our offices every day can be avoided—or at least delayed—by simply preventing damaged skin in the first place. We address this issue in the first part of the program, which is designed for those in their twenties, who are the best candidates for learning things like proper nutrition for healthy skin and the importance of using sunscreen sooner rather than later.
2. **Procedures.** No program would be complete without proactive recommendations, and that's what the procedures portion of the program is. During the middle phase of the program—and, coincidentally, your life—we suggest various surgical and nonsurgical procedures to address the problem areas we've already described throughout this book. The procedures can include lasers and injectables as well as various lifts and tucks or—our preference—a winning combination of the two.
3. **Maintenance.** Finally, as you make your way through your fifties and beyond, we suggest various ways to maintain

and protect the luster and timelessness of your skin that you've worked so hard to achieve in steps 1 and 2. Although these do include several surgical and nonsurgical procedures, we like to think of the maintenance phase as coming full circle to align nicely with the prevention phase. That is, much of the maintenance can be achieved by yourself, at home, using various lotions, potions, and protections to keep your skin looking youthful well into your golden years.

This is not some get-pretty-quick fad or program that is designed for immediate but unrealistic results. This is not us plugging our own line of beauty products or even, for that matter, our services. We don't sell the Beverly Hills Beauty Program T-shirts, flip-flops, key rings, or backpacks. This is simply us offering you our experience in a concise way that will help you to look and feel younger—at any age.

The generational regimen of the Beverly Hills Beauty Program is essentially what most of the stars whom you see in the movies and on television do to keep looking their best. This includes the stars who you and your friends think have *never* had any surgery! This includes the savvy celebrity who does not *want* you to think that they have had any work done. The Beverly Hills Beauty Program is the typical route to achieve that goal.

You, too, can start the program anytime you like; it's never too late or too early. The best part is that it's a very simple combination of our most basic procedures, so there's not a lot to remember. It's simple enough to recall, without the book in hand, and share with your friends and family over lunch or dinner, yet it's thorough enough to solve most of the age-related issues we deal with in our offices on a daily basis.

The age boundaries are a little fuzzy, however. For instance, the advice we offer to those of you in your twenties—wear sunscreen, eat right, practice preventive maintenance—can easily apply to those in their teens as well as those beyond the twenties.

Likewise, the maintenance program we introduce to those of you in your fifties can go well beyond your sixties and even your seventies. The maintenance phase is particularly helpful for those who want to look timeless. The Beverly Hills Beauty Program is really a program for life, and it includes the following:

- **What to do in your twenties.** This is a time for arming yourself against the arrows that Mother Nature eventually slings your way. Since you don't typically have visible signs of aging during your twenties, this is mostly a time when you should be thinking about the damage that is inevitable based on our modern lifestyles. We begin with plenty of education about preventive skin care, including lotions and potions plus microdermabrasion and the use of nonablative lasers to prevent aging and reduce the appearance of fine lines and roughness.

- **What to do in your thirties.** This is when the face (particularly for Caucasians) starts to actively age in ways that are both noticeable and frustrating. Action is key. We fill the bill with Botox as prevention or treatment—including our patented Azizzadeh-Hamilton Conservative Botox (AHCB) approach (for actors who wish to maintain facial movement)—combined with fillers, an active skin-care regimen, and fractional lasers to reverse the signs of aging.

- **What to do in your forties.** Be prepared to consider your first procedure; various procedures will become like friends to you during this critical phase as we smooth and sculpt a face that blends youthfulness with maturity in a way that few will ever notice. The procedures include Thermage, blepharoplasty (eyelid lift), volume restoration with fillers (Perlane, Juvéderm, Radiesse, Sculptra) and/or multilevel fat grafting, and perhaps all the above plus other surgical procedures.

- **What to do in your fifties (and beyond).** This is the time to correct the past and prepare for the future. During your fifties you are introduced to a combined regimen of surgical and nonsurgical procedures, which include all the above restorative measures plus various face-lift approaches to subtly smooth and sculpt your face in preparation for the coming years.

Regardless of your skin tone, color, or texture, the ideas we put forth are sound wisdom culled from treating every kind of case and every kind of face. We are putting forth the way that Hollywood stars erase age and restore youth through the three proven steps of prevention, procedures, and maintenance, to last a lifetime.

Our step-by-step, how-to program is for looking younger, feeling better, and being prouder of your face than you've ever been before. Like most things that are good for you, it all starts with

NOT EVERYBODY TAKES THE DOCTOR'S ADVICE—EVEN IN BEVERLY HILLS

Not long ago, a well-known soap opera star shocked many by going out in public (way) too soon after some obvious cosmetic work. Neither of us treated her at any time, but looking at the pictures on various gossip Web sites, we had to agree that even though the procedures had been done well, it was the actress's insistence on going out in public too soon that caused all the ruckus. It was not a "plastic surgery nightmare," as some sites claimed, or merely shoddy work. We always tell people to take a generous amount of recovery time for each procedure, but it's up to them to follow the doctor's orders. Obviously, celebrities are no different from anyone else in doing or not doing that.

Of course, before the advent of the paparazzi and such tabloid Web sites, people were free to roam around Rodeo Drive at will—before, during, and after surgery—without fear of being "outed" for this procedure or that. Obviously, this has all changed. Now celebrities must exit through rear doors, frequently into alleys where a ride awaits.

With the advent of such Web sites as TMZ.com and www .awfulplasticsurgery.com, every photograph of every celebrity who is even *suspected* of having had some work done can be carefully catalogued, compared, and contrasted to expose just who has had what—and even when. Such sites are indicative of the push-and-pull messages we hear all the time: Is plastic surgery good or bad? As we've mentioned throughout this book, words like *good* and *bad* are judgments made by others, not those of us in the cosmetic rejuvenation industry. It's up to you to decide what you want to have done, not some celebrity or, heaven forbid, gossip Web site!

what you can do—right now—to prevent damage well before Mother Nature does her inevitable dirty work.

The Best Defense Is a Good Offense: Starting Preventive Measures Early

No matter where you are in life, the time to start caring for your skin is right now. Preferably, you should start early in life. We are blessed to have a wonderful actress as a patient whose children already prevent harmful damage to their skin and faces by not only wearing sunscreen and avoiding sun exposure but also using a variety of homeopathic remedies—some of which the actress whips up herself.

Although we urge caution in experimenting with your face, we do applaud this woman for starting her children down the road to healthy skin sooner rather than later. Another celebrity patient never makes an appointment for herself without making one for her teenage daughter as well. Each receives a different treatment, appropriate to her age, and both are showing a proactive interest in reversing the signs of aging—sooner *and* later.

To them, to all our patients, and now to you, we recommend the following advice for starting skin-care prevention as early as possible.

Nutrition Is Nothing "Nu"

Your skin is the largest organ in your body. Because of this, it requires proper nutrition to function optimally, just as all the other organs in your body do. If someone is sick or run-down, you may notice bags under his or her eyes and premature wrinkling.

Your body needs complete nutrition to promote healthy, younger-looking skin. Essential fatty acids help your skin to stay soft and assist in damage repair. About 60 percent of all Americans do not receive enough of these essential fatty acids, which are most commonly found in fish. Dry, itchy, scaly skin is a sign of this deficiency. Vitamins A, C, and E and zinc are also essential to help your skin fight infection and promote healing.

You can help your skin to achieve its optimal health by eating a diet rich in fruits, vegetables, and essential fatty acids. Scientists have found that those who consume foods with plenty of antioxidants and who avoid butter, red meat, and sugar are less prone to wrinkles and enjoy more youthful, vibrant skin.

Sunscreen: Armor in a Tube

We recommend sunscreen to everyone, all the time, *every* time—no excuses! (See the section on sunscreens in chapter 4 for the specifics.) Our philosophy is simple: it's never too early and it's never too late. If you're in your twenties, it's great to get in the habit of wearing sunscreen as often as possible to avoid damage in the future and reduce the chance of skin cancer. With our own children, we have used photo-protective clothing as much as possible and zinc-based sunscreen in exposed regions from infancy.

If you're in your thirties and forties, it's not too late to catch up and build strong habits based on maturity and knowledge as you begin to confront some of the minor damage that may have already been done.

If you're in your fifties and beyond, what are you waiting for? Not only will wearing sunscreen prevent future damage; protecting and preserving your skin at an advanced age allows it to recuperate from the damage done in the past. When you think about it, there really is no good reason *not* to wear sunscreen, just like there is no good reason not to quit smoking.

Nevertheless, sunscreen is only one part of a comprehensive sun-protection regimen. It should be accompanied by other preventive measures, such as the following:

* Avoid being directly in the sun for extended periods (and especially between ten o'clock in the morning and three o'clock in the afternoon)
* Apply sunscreen every four hours. Use a total block that contains zinc, Mexoryl, or Helioplex.

- Choose a sunscreen that is oil-free and not comedogenic (not acne-producing)
- Avoid tanning beds

Maintaining Your Youthful Appearance through the Decades: A Fifty-Year Plan

Whether you start our Beverly Hills Beauty Program today or tomorrow or recommend it to your daughter or your grandmother, it can be implemented at any age and in any situation. It's simple, effective, and clear, just like the specific anti-aging remedies we recommend.

What to Do in Your Twenties: It's Never Too Early to Care for Your Skin

Ah, to be twenty again: youthful skin, radiant appearance, lustrous tone, and vibrant quality. Why is this wondrous, lustrous decade included in the Beverly Hills Beauty Program? The effects of aging are inevitable; we'll all feel them, see them, and experience them at some point—perhaps sooner rather than later. It's important to prevent aging when we can, and there's no better time to do that than at the beginning.

The most important aspect of the twenties phase of the program is prevention. It's not so much about the big, grand things that we do once a month or twice a year, it's about the small, basic, routine decisions we make every single day to care for our skin and prevent damage later. Skin-care products are particularly important because you can use them every single day to either prevent damage or maintain your youthful appearance before, during, and after more serious procedures.

Skin-care products are particularly important because you can use them every single day to either prevent damage or maintain your youthful appearance before, during, and after more serious procedures.

Microdermabrasion can be useful in your twenties. See chapter 5 for a discussion of this procedure. There is very little reason to have aggressive skin treatments in your twenties; skin creams and preventive sun protection are sufficient. We do see many young stars who undergo laser hair reduction and laser treatments for spider veins, however.

What to Do in Your Thirties: Preventive Maintenance Is the Key

The thirties are a magical, marvelous time in terms of skin care and anti-aging. Not only are you at the crest of a youthful wave that has kept your face fairly youthful through your twenties, you are also old enough and wise enough to adopt a prevention program and maintenance through your forties and beyond.

It is, however, a time in which minor aging changes begin to pop up: skin discolorations, fine lines, facial volume loss, and minor drooping. As such, we see many, many people in their thirties who are looking for prevention as well as for treatment of subtle aging changes.

For this reason, the second phase of the Beverly Hills Beauty Program addresses the more noninvasive features of our many treatment options, such as Botox, other fillers and injectables, and lasers. (For a discussion of lasers, see chapter 5.)

Botox: It's Not Just for Foreheads Anymore

In addition to smoothing wrinkles, Botox injections have been known to alleviate migraines, overactive bladders, and Bell's palsy (paralysis of the facial nerve). The injections are also being tested for relief from arthritis and stroke. Officially approved to treat forehead lines, Botox injections are now used off-label to treat a variety of conditions.

Physicians effectively use the treatment to do the following:

- Smooth out horizontal lines on the forehead
- Lift and shape the eyebrows
- Balance asymmetrical features

Another condition being studied is migraines. Studies pioneered by Dr. William Binder, a facial plastic surgeon in Beverly

Hills, suggest that Botox injections can offer relief from chronic headaches, tension headaches, and migraines. The injections have been shown to cause a decrease in the occurrence and severity of migraine headaches for about three to four months after treatment.

The Azizzadeh-Hamilton Conservative Botox Approach

Not long ago we were talking to a patient about nutrition, suggesting various healthy breakfasts, lunches, and dinners. A few days later he came back and was excited about having discovered instant oatmeal for breakfast (rather than his usual fast-food sausage, egg, and bacon burrito at a drive-through on the way to work).

This was a big break for him, but what was even more exciting was that because he found the packets of instant oatmeal too sweet—honey and brown sugar, apples and cinnamon, peaches and cream—he searched until he found a reduced-sugar version so that he could still get the taste he wanted but feel less guilty about it.

That's a little—actually, a lot—like the way we came up with our Azizzadeh-Hamilton Conservative Botox (AHCB) approach. We often work with celebrities who would not be satisfied with a standard Botox treatment. They must have a full range of motion in their mouths, their eyes, their brows, and their cheeks; they must be able to express themselves verbally and visually; and they need a doctor to understand and address this issue with a different kind of Botox treatment.

AHCB is a more conservative dosage of Botox (which we sometimes refer to as "micro-Botox") combined with a more pinpoint precision in placement. The patient would still have the capacity for expressive movement, which is essential for working actors.

AHCB utilizes multiple micro-Botox injections to soften the muscle activity around the eyes without completely paralyzing this region of the face. For instance, in typical Botox injections, four or five injection sites are used on the forehead, with two or three units per site (in large doses). With AHCB, we utilize eight to ten injection sites, with one unit per site (in minimal doses).

In using this method, our celebrity clients can retain their youth and vitality without their appearance going through drastic changes and without losing their range of motion in emotional expressiveness. Furthermore, the risks of Botox are minimized due to the lower dosage.

Fillers and Injectables

Earlier in this book we addressed the subject of how various fillers and injectables can either delay or, in some cases, even replace more serious surgical procedures. The list of items that fillers and injectables can prevent dovetails nicely with the symptoms of aging that are usually experienced in the thirties.

Injectables, which are the main materials used in a liquid face-lift, can treat the following:

- Lost fullness
- Expression lines
- Flattened or hollowed features

After an examination, you and your physician will draw up a treatment plan designed specifically for your signs of aging and your personal goals. This is a critical phase, and we strongly urge you to use all of the information you've gained while reading this book to go into your initial consultation as prepared as possible.

Fillers are probably the main reason that today's Hollywood stars maintain a supple and beautiful appearance throughout their careers. Which fillers do the celebrities like? All of them! They love fillers because they have minimal downtime with subtle but powerful results. Radiesse, Restylane, and Juvéderm are on top of the filler list for most stars; however over the past couple of years, Sculptra has been requested more and more because the results are so gradual.

What to Do in Your Forties: Now Is the Winter of Our Discontent

The forties are traditionally a time of self-evaluation and self-discovery. As we reach the midlife point, it is only natural to look back on what we've accomplished before looking forward to what we have left to do. It is only human nature that we pay a few extra visits to the mirror during this phase of periodic self-examination.

The forties mean different things to different people. Some people are visiting us for the first time. Others are well into the rejuvenation lifestyle and are familiar faces around the office. Still others are halfway through a multiyear program that is designed to help them age fluidly through their forties and beyond.

All the above categories include a list of recognizable celebrities who consider these regimens as required rather than optional. Certain ages are frequently seen by people as milestones that dictate certain procedures. This, of course, might not be warranted.

With all cosmetic procedures, the choice is a personal one. In this section we will discuss how the face ages through the forties and suggest the specific tools you'll need to avoid looking older while you still feel so young.

Nonsurgical Tightening Devices

Nonsurgical skin tightening can be a great way to improve early laxity that is often seen during your forties. We discussed Thermage and other tightening devices in detail in chapter 7.

There are multiple tightening devices on the market that have shown great promise. We believe that in the next ten years, this area of aesthetic medicine will produce even more advanced devices with more reliable results.

Volume Restoration

Volume restoration will be your biggest ally in facing the rigors of time as you make your way through your forties. This is

RED-CARPET BEAUTY SECRETS

Pasadena has the Rose Bowl, Miami has the Dolphins, Seattle has the Sky Needle, and New York has the Empire State Building. What does Beverly Hills have? You might think it's Rodeo Drive or the Beverly Hills Hotel, but you'd be wrong: we've got the Oscars! The awards ceremony itself is right up the street in Hollywood, but where do you think all the stars come for their red-carpet beauty secrets?

The week of the Oscars, and in the months leading up to them, Beverly Hills practically shuts down to accommodate the A-list celebrities and their every beauty need. From salons and stylists to makeup artists and designers, every Beverly Hills specialist is booked months in advance.

Plastic surgeons and dermatologists are no different. Every year, in the months before the Academy Awards, business surges as much as 20 percent. It starts in November and December, when people schedule face-lifts and eyelid lifts that require weeks to heal. The demand for in-office treatments, some of which heal in a matter of hours, picks up in late January.

What are people looking for? They typically come in and say, "I really want to look fresh." They can't go through surgery in that time, so they just want more of a quick-fix type of procedure.

Although we can't divulge the names of the celebrities we've worked on for months, weeks, days, or even minutes before they walked down the ultimate red carpet, we can share their red-carpet beauty secrets with you here.

- **Beauty secret 1: Use what's available.** When you're in a hurry is the wrong time to be trying something absolutely new for you. The best thing our celebrity clients do is to find out what works for them and then use it consistently. For instance, one celebrity sprays her very well-known face with a mixture of water and whole milk in order to keep her famously lustrous skin hydrated throughout the day. Another keeps her face looking fresh by using only lemon juice and water as a homemade astringent. For a new pimple the night before the big day, one celebrity client swears by smoothing toothpaste over the blemish for overnight relief. You'll never know what works for you until you try; we suggest starting with the three red-carpet beauty secrets just mentioned. And never forget to include a top drawer make-up artist and hair stylist as part of your team.

- **Beauty secret 2: Timing is everything.** Don't do too much too soon—but do as much as you can in the time you have allotted. Do you have two months to recover, or two weeks? Depending on the length of your recovery time, you will have to choose which procedures are right for you. Discuss with your physician when the event will be and how much time you'll need to recover; then decide how much or how little you can afford to get done.

- **Beauty secret 3: Less is more.** For your own red-carpet event—be it a wedding, an awards ceremony, a charity event, or your wedding anniversary—remember that the secret to looking A-list glamorous is less, not more. Now is *not* the time to be considering major surgery, or even nonsurgical procedures with long recovery times.

- **Beauty secret 4: Accentuate the positive.** Your face is only one part of the first impression that you make. As you use new beauty products or sample these red-carpet beauty secrets, don't neglect to get your hair done. If you color it, do so in enough time for it to look natural on your big day. Think about what makeup you'll wear, down to the shade of lipstick or the severity of your blush. If you want a tan, make sure that you do that spray tan the correct number of days in advance. Even accessories should be planned out in advance. Why do you think most of Beverly Hills shuts down in the weeks before Oscar night? Everybody's running from store to store, trying to accessorize!

- **Beauty secret 5: The AHCB approach.** Directors don't like an actor's face to be expressionless; nor should you want *your* face to be that way. Suggest that your physician incorporate some form of our AHCB approach, which is essentially just a more conservative dosage of Botox along with precision targeting of the appropriate muscle regions. The patient can still make expressive facial movements, which is especially important for working actors but just as desirable for anyone else who doesn't want to look like a mannequin.

typically when we see people who are on their very first visit to a dermatologist or a plastic surgeon.

Few consider the damage done during their thirties—and others simply ignore it—but when the forties strike, that's when people really start to notice the wrinkles around their eyes, the furrowing of their brows, the drooping of their eyelids, or the weakness of their chins.

Volume loss is one of the main culprits in aging at this time, resulting in hollowness and exacerbating the sagging process that is also in motion. Hence, by restoring the volume to the face, we can both rectify the problem and temporarily eliminate, or at least delay, the need for more extensive procedures. We often have to point out that the cheeks will be made full, not fat; the latter is an unwarranted concern.

There are two prevailing treatments for volume loss that are both safe and effective face-lift alternatives: the filler liquid face-lift and multilevel fat grafting (MFG). See chapter 7 for a full discussion of these methods.

Surgical Procedures

We have learned that all faces age differently. Some stay smooth and supple well into the forties and beyond, whereas others change texture and fullness while their "owners" are still in their thirties. You can compare this to hair loss: some lose their hair prematurely, whereas others keep a full head of hair well into their senior years.

Unlike hair loss, however, not all facial aging is hereditary. Sun and your own behaviors can contribute to a face's aging well before its time. Some of you may therefore need more vigorous procedures in your forties than others do. Blepharoplasty (eyelid lift) and the brow lift are the most commonly performed operations on the Hollywood celebrities in this age group, because the eyes and the surrounding regions tend to be the first to show their age. Ultimately, it's up to you and your doctor to determine how much is necessary, if any, and how soon.

It's very, very difficult to hide aging in the eyes. Depending on the specific program, any one or more of the following procedures may be needed: blepharoplasty, fillers, laser resurfacing, or more complex surgeries. Once again, analysis of the problem is key to the final outcome. See chapter 8 for a full discussion of the surgical procedures.

What to Do in Your Fifties and Beyond: Bring in the Reinforcements!

The fifties are a magical time for modern men and women who want to remain looking youthful as they age. More and more often these days, you hear that sixty is the new fifty or that fifty is the new forty. We can tell you that it's (mostly) true, particularly for our celebrity clients, who look more youthful now than their noncelebrity peers do.

As more and more women *and* men use beauty products to slow the process of aging in their twenties, thirties, and forties, the fifty-year-olds we see now look more like the forty-year-olds we saw twenty and thirty years ago.

Even so, Mother Nature is not so easily fooled, and the fifties are still a time of major changes in the texture, laxity, and fullness of your skin. To address these very age-specific conditions, we have combined a series of very age-specific remedies.

Various Face-Lift Approaches

To maintain a youthful appearance throughout your fifties and beyond, remember the "neighborhood" of your face. From forehead to chin, a qualified physician will help you to address the problems you have now and/or might face in the future.

Remember the various lift procedures that are available to you, and, if necessary, reread the chapters that address them in order to help you better understand what is right for you. We discussed the following four types of lifts:

- Brow or forehead lift
- Eyelid lift
- Cheek or midface-lift

- Face-lift (lower face)
- Neck lift

Maintenance: Follow the "Five-Finger" Approach

Looking back on the advice we've given you throughout this book, we believe that we've made a strong case for personal accountability. It is, after all, your face that we're talking about here. What we can do, we'll do; what products and procedures can do, they'll do. You, however, must be part of the equation as well.

We all know people who have a daily regimen of skin care. We've even shared with you our own recommendations for rejuvenating actions. What do you actually *do*, morning, noon, and night, to reverse age and welcome restoration? If you don't know—or haven't yet decided—this is the time to figure it out.

In the fifties and beyond, you are in the critical phase of aging. We don't mean to sound too alarmist, but this is when the rubber really hits the road in terms of seeing the effects of aging across a spectrum of wrinkle, laxity, and texture issues.

Just as we have provided a comprehensive approach to combining surgery with fillers or lasers with lifts, so too must you settle into a routine maintenance regimen, not only to protect whatever procedures you've had done, but also to maintain the appearance of youthfulness and fullness between procedures.

This doesn't affect just your appearance; it affects your pocketbook as well. The more maintenance you do between office visits, the fewer procedures you will have to have done when you do pay us a visit. Maintenance doesn't have to take all day—or all of your budget. In fact, we suggest the "five-finger" approach to enlisting the help of beauty products in your daily maintenance routine.

In short, keep it simple, remember that less is more, and stay within a range of five helpful products—one to remember on each of your fingers. Timeless skin care includes the five following rules:

1. Cleanse
2. Exfoliate
3. Moisturize
4. Tone
5. Protect

By following the five-finger approach, you have a product that works for each of the above rules. This means that you should have the following:

1. A quality soap that works for your skin and your budget. This is your staple, the one you use night and day for gentle cleaning. It satisfies the *cleanse* rule.
2. A light astringent for when deep cleaning is necessary, such as after a day in the garden or a tough workout. This will help to increase blood flow and remove excess surface oils to help establish a clean/glowing look.
3. A quality moisturizer to help keep your skin radiant; this satisfies the *moisture* rule.
4. A quality lotion to help you keep your skin *toned* and beautiful. There are many quality lotions and potions on the market, including products that are full of antioxidants and hydroxy acids.
5. A daily routine to protect your skin, usually in the morning and at night. This should include a broad-spectrum (UVB and UVA blocker) sunscreen with zinc, an SPF of 15 or higher, and Mexoryl or Helioplex in the morning and a restorative cream or gel at night to repair facial damage while you sleep.

By keeping your maintenance routine and supplies simple, you are much more likely to actually use them. The five-finger approach is all about simplicity and effectiveness. We want to keep it simple because, in our experience, people tend to do the bare minimum; so if your bare minimum is to use the five best products on the market to clean, exfoliate, moisturize, tone, and protect your skin every day, then that's what we want you to do.

Even the stars follow our five-finger approach. Despite having enough money to live in a spa and enough time to exfoliate

24/7, these beautiful, glamorous, and youthful-looking men and women still tend to do the same five things every morning and every evening to maintain youthful, healthy-looking skin.

These are people whose faces are often their livelihood. They tend to stick with what works, and what works is often the best products on the market used twice daily to clean, exfoliate, moisturize, tone, and protect.

You should also be on the lookout for new products to add to your routine: a new cleanser that's gentler on your skin—or

CELEBRITIES WHO'VE DONE IT ALL WRONG

It is very unfortunate when *any* corrective procedure goes wrong, but it's especially painful when the whole world is watching, which is what happens when celebrities have bad plastic surgery.

In our modern tabloid-rampant culture, every stitch, nip, and tuck is on display for the world to see. How would we feel if our old yearbook photos from the 1950s, 1960s, and 1970s were put side by side with pictures of us today? How would it look if someone took a quick snapshot of us and blew it up to twice its size to expose scar tissue around the neck, breasts, or belly button? Unfortunately, this kind of intense media scrutiny, which is what celebrities go through, would be a difficult situation for anyone.

Nevertheless, even though thousands of celebrities, musicians, artists, and politicians have plastic surgery, there has been only a handful of botched operations. It is hard to know what went wrong. Obviously, bad decisions can be made by either the surgeon or the patient.

On more than one occasion, celebrities who have had good work done by other surgeons have come into our office because they are unhappy with the results, due to either a pathologically skewed body image (body dysmorphic disorder) or unreasonable expectations. It is our job to educate them about the possible good and bad effects of fillers and/or surgery. Sometimes they listen, and, unfortunately, sometimes they don't.

even your pocketbook; a new moisturizer that's more organic than what you used to use; an exfoliant that brings new life to your face.

Don't let the learning process end with the last page of this book; continue to ask your dermatologist or facial plastic surgeon for recommendations, scan women's magazines, search your favorite beauty products Web site, and even watch TV to continue to learn about beauty products that not only work well but work for you. Most important, get feedback from your physician about your purchases.

10

How to Choose a Doctor

The 95 Percent Factor

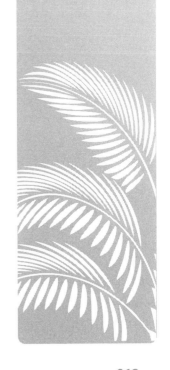

*P*icture this: A pregnant woman comes into an obstetrician's office to have her baby delivered. She enters an exam room, and in comes a gentleman dressed in a white lab coat. However, underneath his lab coat, he is wearing a cab driver's uniform. If you were that pregnant woman, would you go ahead with the delivery under those circumstances?

In 95 percent of the cases, it's actually just as safe to have your baby delivered by a cab driver—or anyone else, for that matter—as by a highly trained and board-certified obstetrician. Medical students with very little experience, next-door neighbors with *no* experience, and almost anyone who comes along (including a cab driver) at just the right time, under just the right conditions, can "catch" a baby as well as an obstetrician can. Yet very few pregnant women would stop going to the obstetrician, because of that slim—perhaps 5 percent chance—of problems or complications.

This is what we call the *95 percent factor*.

For the same reason, cosmetic procedures—either invasive or noninvasive—that are performed by individuals who are not trained and certified by one of the five core cosmetic specialties (dermatology, facial plastic surgery, plastic surgery, oculoplastic surgery, or otolaryngology), run the same risk of the 5 percent harm factor as the woman who would have her baby delivered by a cab driver instead of an obstetrician.

Who are these noncertified doctors, and where are these nonclinical settings? If you've ever received a brochure from a cheerily smiling man in a lab coat who is offering serious cosmetic procedures whose names are accompanied by asterisks (or seen this same type of fellow on a billboard or on the side of a bus as you drive or walk through town), chances are you've just met a noncertified doctor. If you've ever driven by a chain salon, spa, or beauty parlor that offers laser hair removal and chemical peels while you're getting your nails done or your feet massaged, you've seen what we in the trade refer to as a *nonclinical* setting.

These days, an alarming number of serious cosmetic procedures are being performed at an increasing array of nonclinical, or off-site, locations all across the country; they range from beauty parlors to nail salons to day spas, where individuals can get procedures ranging from laser resurfacing to chemical peels to injectables like Botox.

We realize that the Web sites, brochures, billboards, and print ads can be enticing. How great would it be to have a serious medical procedure performed in a nonclinical setting while you're being treated to a foot massage, a steam bath, or a mud-soak treatment? All the while, dim lighting, aromatherapy candles, and nature CDs playing in the background set the mood and ease your fears. It *would* be great—that is, if the physicians doing the treatments were all board-certified—or, for that matter, if they were even physicians.

The problem is that there is too much of a good thing being performed by too many people with bad qualifications. Modern technology has given many in this country a license to perform medical procedures that didn't exist three or four years ago using products that sometimes weren't around even last year—all in the hands of relative novices.

As a matter of fact, as little as five years ago, *we* weren't doing 80 percent of the procedures we're doing today; technology has opened up a veritable Pandora's box for providers and consumers, not to mention physicians—or those who would call themselves physicians. Today, everybody thinks that he or she can handle a laser or inject Botox. There has been a tidal wave of nonprofessionals who are providing services all across the country, from beauty parlors and nail technicians to noncertified doctors who are offering outpatient services in a variety of nonmedical settings.

People often think it's cheaper to get these procedures done at a spa or a salon, but such work may in fact be more expensive there than in a clinical setting with a board-certified specialist. Someone has to pay for all that ambiance—the friendly staff, the pretty pink lab coats, the exotic mud baths, and the pricey candles—yet expensive marketing and advertising makes the opposite seem true.

You're also paying for all that advertising, in the form of similar or slightly higher fees for the same procedures that we can give you safely, carefully, efficiently, and clinically. Chains build themselves by making more money than the competitors and expanding their business base by opening more stores to make more money—and on and on it goes.

We're all in favor of day spas or salons that offer a variety of services that the practitioners are qualified to perform, but to offer medical procedures as well is akin to selling hardware at a fruit stand; one of these things is not like the other, and it can be very damaging in the long run. Of course, the draw of salons is not really safety or even cost; it's the frou frou environment—softer, less clinical, and with a soothing ambiance, unlike what is typically found in a doctor's office. The salon can feel more welcoming and less frightening—but is it safer?

Such is the appeal of Botox parties; even though you're getting a medical procedure done, the party atmosphere, with its wine and smiles and good fellowship, makes you feel as if you're at just another party. The same is true for a salon atmosphere; in addition to getting pink lighting, New Age music, and aromatherapy candles, you're also getting a clinical procedure.

You can expect many things at a spa or a salon: pleasant lighting, fast service, and a welcoming atmosphere. However, *you* will still have to make sure that a qualified medical professional is actually performing the procedures. Beauty parlors, salons, and day spas make you feel as if the procedure you're having is no more serious than a permanent or a pedicure. Is that a reality? Think about it: you're having a toxin injected into your face, highly sensitive chemicals slathered on it, and/or lasers scanning your delicate dermal layer (which can produce burns). Is that really the same as styling your hair or polishing your nails?

We're certainly not trying to be alarmists here; as the 95 percent factor indicates, 95 percent of the time there aren't any problems, serious or otherwise, with the procedures that are done in these settings. Furthermore, some of the physicians (whether board-certified or not) who perform the procedures in these places are ethical doctors who are practicing appropriately. Our only concern is that 5 percent of the time, we *do* see problems—and serious ones—as a result of these over-the-counter cosmetic procedures.

Some (not all) of the physicians or nurses who are performing procedures at these places have not been trained well enough or long enough to know what the risks are, and they certainly do not know how to handle problems that *do* arise during the procedure. All the aromatherapy candles and mud baths in the world won't save your face from an inexperienced physician who is botching a procedure that is well outside his or her purview—and who has no medical staff on-site for backup.

In the final analysis, the 95 percent factor is similar to the reality for commercial airline pilots when they fly: 95 percent of the time, the plane is on automatic pilot. You or I could do that part, but would you consider going into the cockpit and taking over the plane for the entire flight? Would you want one of your fellow passengers to do the same? Certainly not, and the same goes for letting someone work on your face who is not appropriately trained to do so.

Most of the spa settings that are becoming popular do not even have a supervising physician on the premises. In many cases, the supervising physician hasn't been on the premises in days, weeks, or months. Worse than that, the supervising physicians are sometimes not even specialists in the core cosmetic specialties; they are merely physicians whose license is being used by the owners of the spas to generate an income. This is quite a different setting from what a registered nurse or a physician's assistant can provide in the appropriate medical setting with a well-trained physician as his or her supervisor.

The spa phenomenon also feeds a psychological element that is rarely addressed: a patient's anxiety in coming to a physician's office with its very clinical environment. Spas provide an illusion of pseudosurgical support and pampering, something between a beauty salon and a vacation resort. What the customer should always remember, however, is that lasers and injections are medical procedures, not cosmetics. If your new hairdo is bad, it lasts a month; if your face is damaged, it could last much longer and at a much greater cost.

You don't have to drive by a strip mall salon that's offering laser resurfacing or come across an ad for "quick and inexpensive Botox injections" in your local paper to see the pitfalls of the 95 percent factor. Just turn on the nightly news; recent developments here in Hollywood have illustrated the danger of the 95 percent factor, when botched surgeries and even death are the result of dangerous procedures performed by inexperienced or unscrupulous physicians.

It is possible that in the future there will be a proliferation of public outings of so-called famous dermatologists and "celebrity" plastic surgeons, in which they are revealed to have no board certification or qualifications for the procedures that they have been providing for years, many of them on national TV. Although many will be surprised by such developments, we won't. That's because board certification is an ethical and a professional qualification, not a mandatory one. By law, one merely has to be a licensed physician—in any field—to perform myriad procedures with a variety of products with which many doctors have had little or no training. We often hear of general practitioners who do face-lifts or pediatricians who specialize in microdermabrasion—because, quite simply, there's nothing and no one to stop them. A family doctor or a pediatrician could perform brain surgery and it would be legal!

Therefore, if you have a public that doesn't understand the laws and bylaws of board certification, let alone state licensing, and you combine that with a bevy of new products and procedures that are released every year along with an affordable and seemingly safe alternative in over-the-counter procedures performed in nonmedical settings, what you get is complete miscommunication, misrepresentation, and misuse that often result in less than stellar, if not outright dangerous, outcomes.

It's not all doom and gloom out there; there are many board-certified physicians all over the country who provide excellent care. We are simply pointing out that your procedures should be attended to by physicians with these entry-level qualifications—at a bare minimum, board certification—which reduce your chances of being in the 5 percent of people who wind up with bad results. Even when you *are* dealing with a board-certified physician, you should still do your homework. There are a few board-certified physicians who are simply poor physicians.

In other words, "let the buyer beware." You have to investigate whether a physician has had residency training and board certification in a procedure. (We show you how to do this in the next chapter.) That is the responsibility of the patient, unfortunately, at this time in the United States. Should the regulations be otherwise? We'll leave that up to you to decide.

The Final Word on Board Certification

Here is a surprising fact: Most people believe that in order to call yourself a dermatologist, a plastic surgeon, or a cosmetic surgeon, you must have received specialized medical training, residency training (of three to six years), and board certification. Nothing could be farther from the truth.

The only requirement for calling yourself a practitioner of one of those specialties is to have a medical license; this means that you have to have completed an internship—only one year beyond medical school—to call yourself any of those titles. Furthermore, some physicians do actually complete residency training in one of the core cosmetic specialties, but they do not pass the requirements of the boards and fail to become board-certified; thus, although these physicians would generally be better qualified to treat you than one who has never had any specialty training in one of the core specialties, they are not actually certified to do so. We will describe here the five different specialists and the credentials they should have.

Dermatologists are certified by the American Board of Dermatology. After medical school, dermatologists typically undergo one year of internship followed by three years of dermatology residency. Dermasurgeons are dermatologists with special interests and expertise in skin surgery and noninvasive cosmetic procedures such as fillers and lasers. Dermasurgeons are members of the American Society of Dermatologic Surgery. Some dermasurgeons are skilled in performing procedures outside their core training, for example, face lifts and eyelid surgeries.

PROCEDURES AND THE APPROPRIATE BOARD-CERTIFIED PHYSICIAN

We urge our readers to review the list of certifying organizations—"How to Know Your Doctor Knows (Is He or She Up-to-Date?)"—in chapter 2.

Noninvasive facial rejuvenation: injectables and lasers

- Dermatologist
- Facial plastic surgeon
- Plastic surgeon
- Oculoplastic surgeon

Face-lift

- Facial plastic surgeon
- Plastic surgeon

Blepharoplasty

- Facial plastic surgeon
- Plastic surgeon
- Oculoplastic surgeon

Rhinoplasty

- Facial plastic surgeon
- Plastic surgeon

MFG

- Facial plastic surgeon
- Plastic surgeon

Chin and cheek augmentation

- Facial plastic surgeon
- Plastic surgeon

Brow lift

- Facial plastic surgeon
- Plastic surgeon
- Oculoplastic surgeon

Otoplasty (ear reshaping)

- Facial plastic surgeon
- Plastic surgeon

Facial and neck liposuction

- Facial plastic surgeon
- Plastic surgeon

Facial plastic surgeons should be certified by the American Board of Facial Plastic and Reconstructive Surgery as well as the American Board of Otolaryngology, which is recognized by the American Board of Medical Specialties (ABMS). Facial plastic surgeons should also belong to the American Academy of Facial Plastic and Reconstructive Surgery. Facial plastic surgeons typically spend five to six years in postgraduate surgical training in otolaryngology, with a specialty in head and neck surgery, followed by a subspecialty fellowship in facial plastic and reconstructive surgery.

The primary focus of facial plastic surgeons is the cosmetic and reconstructive surgery of the face, the eyes, the neck, and the nose. Concentrating on the complex anatomy, physiology, pathology, and biochemistry of all of the organs and structures of the head and neck provides the facial plastic surgeon with a strong knowledge of that anatomical region.

Plastic surgeons should be certified by the American Board of Plastic Surgery (which also is part of the ABMS) and belong to the American Society for Aesthetic Plastic Surgery. Plastic surgeons typically perform surgery on the entire body, including the face. You should inquire to see if they have any areas of specialty. Plastic surgeons typically have three to seven years of general surgery training followed by two to three years of plastic surgery training.

Oculoplastic surgeons are certified by the American Board of Ophthalmology and belong to the American Society of Ophthalmic Plastic and Reconstructive Surgery. Oculoplastic surgeons perform cosmetic and reconstructive surgery of the eyelids, the orbit (the bony socket of the eye), and associated regions. Ophthalmologists who do not have fellowship training in oculoplastic surgery typically do not have enough expertise in cosmetic eyelid surgery.

Cosmetic surgeon is a generic term that is used by many different specialties. You have to be sure that these practitioners have board certification by one of the abovementioned boards and perform surgeries within their specialties. You don't want a board-certified facial plastic surgeon performing your tummy tuck or an oculoplastic surgeon doing your nose job.

We often hear questions like the following: "I just had Botox done by a board-certified physician who happens to be an orthopedic surgeon. Is that okay?" No, it is *not* okay! We certainly don't mean to bash board-certified orthopedic surgeons, but would you want your spinal surgery performed by a board-certified plastic surgeon? Of course not!

The key is that your board-certified physician has to stick to the areas in which he or she trained. Don't be fooled by physicians who say that they are board-certified; ask them the *specific area* in which they are certified, and make sure that they are performing procedures within that specialty.

Finally, be aware that any organization can create its own boards, so make sure that your specialist belongs to one of the five core specialty boards mentioned above: the American Board of Dermatology, the American Board of Plastic Surgery, the American Board of Facial Plastic and Reconstructive Surgery, the American Board of Otolaryngology, or the American Board of Ophthalmology (with an ophthalmic plastic surgery fellowship).

How to Look for a Facial Rejuvenation Specialist

Choosing the right cosmetic specialist is one of the most important decisions you will make during the process of achieving the more youthful look you desire. It is important that you find a dermatologist or a facial plastic surgeon who is not just competent and experienced in his or her chosen profession, but who understands your individual needs and goals. (We call this the *click factor*, and we'll discuss it a little later in this chapter.) We have put together some general guidelines to help you know what to look for and what to consider when consulting with facial rejuvenation specialists.

The first step will also be the most obvious: where to look. We see ads for plastic surgeons all day long: on the bus, in the mall, on TV, in local newspapers, and in the yellow pages. How do you know if any one of those doctors is the right one for you?

There are several ways to go about making this very serious choice; the following comprehensive list should be helpful in your search for a facial rejuvenation specialist:

- **Ask for a referral.** If you can get a referral from a trusted physician or specialist, we recommend this as a great place to start. This way you are getting a name—or maybe several—from a respected, credentialed physician whom you already trust. The key here is to gather a list of names based on credible sources, not just names that are found on bus benches and in yellow page ads. They might be credible physicians, but visibility and popularity shouldn't be your only two criteria for choosing a physician.

- **Start with your own personal network.** If your doctor can't make a recommendation, reach outside the medical field—but not too far—to ask friends and family or even coworkers you know and trust whom they might recommend. Stick with people who you know have had procedures done and are satisfied with them; speak with them discreetly about whom they used, their satisfaction level, cost, complaints, and so on. Don't go by hearsay alone, however; look to see if the results they have are the same as what you want. For instance, if someone you know has the surprised look that we discussed earlier, you might not want their recommendation in the first place.

- **Narrow down your choices.** Once you've gathered some referrals, begin to build a short list of potential candidates. This could be three to five names, or it could be eight to ten; either way, the shorter your list, the better your chances of gathering more information on each doctor. We suggest writing down each doctor's name at the top of a notebook page and listing all you've learned about him or her. As you continue to do research, write down what you find, and once you're satisfied that you've done all your homework, carefully analyze your findings before ranking the names on your short list. Then begin approaching each doctor, one by one.

- **Go directly to the source.** As you narrow down your short list, first visit the doctor's Web site and confirm the obvious, such as education and board certification (see the Web site addresses in chapter 2). Then you should interview each doctor and specifically ask for his or her credentials (see our list of recommended questions later in this chapter). This is different from an initial consultation about your face. This is a preconsultation to see if you and your potential doctor are compatible. Think of it as a job interview, and you'll get the basic idea.

- **Lather, rinse, repeat.** It might be necessary for you to start your search all over again if your list of candidates falls short in any number of ways (see the "five Cs" below). Don't be discouraged if this occurs. It's better for you to spend more time before your procedure looking for a qualified doctor who'll do it right the first time than to have to repeat the whole process again after the procedure in order to find someone else to clean up a mess.

Malpractice is a huge issue these days, but being sued for malpractice is not grounds for losing one's medical license. After all, in this country, anyone can sue anyone, and only 20 percent of all medical malpractice suits are actually valid.

Nevertheless, if you are being thorough about your research, you will want to find out as much about your potential doctor as is humanly possible, and this naturally includes whether there have been any complaints made against him or her. How do you learn if your doctor has been sued—and why?

Every state has a medical board, and there you can find the information you need. Start by visiting your state's official Web site, where you should be able to easily locate the medical board and find either a searchable database online or the physical contact information you'll need to obtain this information offline as well. You may have to pay a small service fee for the official request, but knowing that your doctor hasn't been sued for medical malpractice is well worth the $5 or $10 application fee, don't you think?

What to Look For in a Doctor: The Five-C Method

In discussing how to look for a specialist, we mentioned the "five Cs" method. When you are choosing a facial rejuvenation doctor, you should look for the following five qualities:

1. **Compassion.** Compassion is at the top of our list because you want a doctor who is going to truly care about your

results, not some paint-by-numbers physician who is just going through the motions. Every face is different, and no face is more important than your own. Don't you want to have someone working on your face who cares about it as much as you do? Locating a doctor and choosing a doctor are two very different things. After all, you wouldn't buy the first house you visit; you'd want to take the full tour, explore every room, test the faucets, open the cabinets—kick the tires, so to speak—and then come back after you've explored every other available option. The same is true of your facial rejuvenation specialist; meet with him or her personally before committing to any procedure, and really trust your gut to guide you on whether he or she is truly the right doctor for you.

2. **Confidence.** You want a doctor who is confident about the work. When the doctor answers your questions, really listen to the responses. Is he or she just throwing around five-dollar words to avoid revealing a lack of knowledge of the answers, or do the responses make sense and, more important, make you feel better about what he or she has just said? Your doctor should know the answers to all of your questions and be able to give you responses that are clear, concise, and confident. If the doctor is hesitant or uncertain, you should be less confident about choosing him or her.

3. **Comprehensiveness.** When you select your physician, make sure that he or she has the knowledge base for all of your facial rejuvenation needs, and in the most comprehensive way. If your physician is a dermatologist, he or she should know when the needle or the laser wouldn't solve your problem and when a surgical specialist should be consulted. On the other hand, many surgeons know how to use the scalpel but have no idea about the importance of skin rejuvenation. Comprehensive facial rejuvenation requires your specialist to know all facets of facial rejuvenation so you get the best possible outcome.

4. **Compatibility.** You want to be very compatible with the person who is working on your face, so make sure that you

and your doctor "click." As mentioned above, we call this the *click factor*. We don't know any other way to put it. It's a subjective opinion, to be sure, but the click factor should be there if you and your doctor are really going to connect on both a personal and a professional level. This doesn't mean that you have to be friends and go out for lunch; it merely means that you understand each other and that he or she is really listening to what you're saying. The click factor is pretty immediate: most people know after a few minutes of speaking with us whether we're going to click. We don't always do so, but what's important to remember about being compatible with your physician is that you must both be yourselves.

5. **Certification.** We really can't stress this enough; use the information provided in the previous section and find a board-certified physician who has expertise in the area of your concern. It takes a little more time, a little more research, and a little more effort, but trust us: it is well worth the exertion. Remember the 95 percent factor; you don't want to be in the 5 percent that experiences trouble as a result of skipping this step and having a very serious procedure done at a location without a board-certified doctor.

What to Ask: The Preconsultation Interview

In chapter 2 we introduced how to go about making the most of the initial consultation with your physician; now we'd like to revisit that discussion and remind you just how vital it is to take this meeting seriously.

Some doctors compare the initial consultation with your facial plastic surgeon or dermatologist to a first date; it's a chance to get to really know each other and feel your way around the conversation. However, we prefer to think of it as more like the night before your wedding; this is no time to be shy about the hard questions. If you're having cold feet, find out why.

Therefore, we have put together this comprehensive guide for you to use when preparing for that all-important initial consultation. You might want to make notes in the margins, photocopy these pages, or even make a list of your own to bring along.

Don't be afraid to ask your doctor questions. We're always thrilled when people come prepared with plenty of questions; not only does it make our jobs easier, it also always makes the procedure go more smoothly in the end. If you sense that the doctor doesn't like being asked questions, then that is a sign that this is not the right doctor for you.

Is the Doctor's Experience Relevant to You?

Of course you want a cosmetic specialist who is experienced. A good cosmetic specialist must not only be experienced in the clinical portions of facial rejuvenation, he or she must also have a strong aesthetic sense and a history of creating optimal and realistic results.

To get a better feel for your physician's work, ask to see examples of some of his or her before and after pictures of actual individuals. Pay particular attention to people who share traits in common with you such as ethnicity, age, facial structure, and any other factors that are important to you. It is this specific experience that is often most directly relevant to you.

Does the Doctor Listen to You?

The capacity to listen goes back to one of the five Cs: compatibility. Even though your cosmetic specialist's previous work can be an excellent indicator of his or her abilities, the most important thing is the quality of work the physician can provide. It is important to choose someone who takes the time to understand your goals and needs.

Talk to your doctor about what results you're looking for, explain your preferences, and be brutally honest about what you expect, not only from yourself but also from your physician.

You will know that you have found the right physician when you feel understood 100 percent.

Who Decides What the Finished Product Will Look Like—You or Your Doctor?

You decide what you want to look like. However, it is up to your doctor to discuss with you how realistic your desires are compared to what products and procedures are currently available to achieve that effect. For instance, you might want a simple face-lift, but your doctor can help you to explore other options instead of or even in addition to a face-lift that will give you an effect beyond what you even considered possible.

Conversely, you may have unrealistic expectations of what exactly your facial rejuvenation expert can achieve. When both of you are open and honest with each other, your initial disappointment can be offset by the fact that the result will be the product of a mutual discussion based on mutual respect.

Although your ideas and expectations are always important, remember that your doctor is a trained professional whose job is to help you achieve those ideas and expectations; by staying up-to-date and informed about various products and procedures, he or she can help to turn your dreams into reality—but only if you let that happen!

Does the Doctor Offer Computer Imaging for Plastic Surgery?

Computer imaging is a great way for both you and your doctor to literally see into the future. By uploading digital photographs of your face during the initial consultation, we can see—in real time and right before our very eyes—how the changes you are looking for will affect your face.

This effectively allows us to try a variety of procedures and view the results before committing to any true physical changes. This is often considered a troubleshooting process in which we can show the patient how less is more in the latest cosmetic procedures.

Sophisticated computer technology allows us to morph your facial features—by adding to or taking away—for a result that produces a "future you" based on present reality. Many of our patients are relieved to be able to see the approximated results of their procedures before actually committing to such procedures. The most common procedures that computer imaging assists with are rhinoplasty, chin augmentation, and neck rejuvenation.

How Much Will You Change as a Result of the Procedure?

The goal of successful cosmetic enhancement is for you to improve the areas with which you are concerned. We just want those changes to be gradual and complementary to your unique and original face. The goal is not to make you look like someone else, but to make you look like yourself—only better.

Nevertheless, there will be change, and you will notice it. Many of your closest friends and family members will also notice something different but may have difficulty saying what it is. We don't want them to notice it too much; that is why we never do too much or too little, but only enough to affect the change you want in a way that is complementary to your face and never severe or too dramatic.

Will You Still Look Like Yourself after the Procedure?

Our ultimate goal is not just for you to look like yourself after the procedure but also for you to look like your best possible self. This is really the goal of any procedure: keeping the true, authentic you intact while trying hard to erase any signs of aging or skin damage that have managed to cloud the old you.

Don't be surprised, however, if people notice the new you after the procedure. Questions like "Did you change your hair?" "Did you just come from the salon?" or even "Have you been on vacation?" are quite common after surgery. We *want* people to notice; don't you?

Final Words about Finding Your Doctor

All we can do in this book is to guide you through the physical motions of locating a facial rejuvenation specialist: how, where, and what to ask. The decision, however, has been, is now, and always will be yours and yours alone.

We hope that this chapter has provided you with more than just the details of how to go about finding a doctor. We have tried to share with you how important your gut instincts are in helping your head to make the right decision.

Remember the click factor; make sure you and your doctor connect. This is something you won't find in a book or on a chart or through a background check, but having compatibility with your doctor is crucial to make sure that you understand each other when you discuss the proper products and procedures during your initial consultation. These are very important decisions that you're making about your face, and you want a doctor who will both listen to your needs and educate you about the realities of the options. In fact, you want your doctor to challenge you a little, because he or she is an expert.

We caution you against finding a "yes" doctor who will merely give you anything you want. In this case, the customer might not always be right, and your doctor can explain why what you've asked for may not be the right thing for you at this time. We'd rather have you be slightly disappointed in your expectations about a procedure in the very beginning if it means that your doctor can give you much better results in the end.

The path to a healthier, more youthful-appearing face is long, and it requires a strong partnership between you and your doctor. Take the time to lay a solid foundation for this critical relationship by doing your research and finding the right doctor for you—not just the easiest doctor to locate. Trust us, your face will thank you!

11

Reading Between the Lines

Questions That Frequently Should Be Asked but Aren't

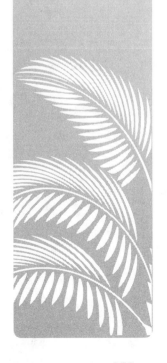

Many books on skin care and plastic surgery end with a section containing their readers' most frequently asked questions, or FAQs; however, this chapter is much more than that. This is not so much a section on answering your questions as it is a practical, user-friendly guide to help *you* ask your physician the right questions.

Questions and answers are the basis for not only a good initial consultation but also a safe and successful procedure. Don't make the mistake of thinking you know too much—or not enough—to ask any questions. If you are uncertain about something even though you *think* you know the answer, ask about it, anyway. If your doctor's reply merely confirms what you already thought you knew, so much the better; now you can feel even more comfortable about the procedure. If you didn't already know what you thought you did, now you *do* know; it's a win-win situation by any stretch of the imagination.

As we have just seen in the previous chapter, it is vital that you ask the physician the right questions at the right times. If he or she can't, or won't, answer them to your satisfaction, then you are well within your rights to seek medical attention elsewhere. Frankly, after all you've read up to this point, we'd be disappointed if you didn't!

Thus, in order to arm you with those questions, we have divided this chapter into the following sections:

- **What to ask (yourself) before the consultation.** Your doctor isn't alone in performing your procedure; you are an equal and willing participant in seeking his or her help. It is therefore important to ask as many questions of yourself *before* your initial consultation as it will be to ask them of your doctor *during* the consultation.

- **What to ask before the procedure.** While you are slipping into a hospital gown or going under from anesthesia is *not* the right time to be asking questions about your procedure. You need to be prepared *before* either of these things happens so that you know exactly what to expect *when* they happen (or, preferably, long before that point). The questions in this section will help to ensure that both you and your doctor are thinking alike.

- **What to ask before you are released.** Many people go home silently, without being prepared for the eventual soreness, bruising, and/or pain that can accompany a procedure. We don't want you to be one of them, so be prepared by reading this section and asking your doctor exactly what to expect before you are released.

Trust us; your doctor wants to help you be prepared for your cosmetic procedure. Unfortunately, with time at a premium and so many patients and procedures coming through the office each week, it is naturally very difficult for every physician to be 100 percent sensitive to every single patient. That is why doctors often rely on you, the patient, to nudge them into giving you every possible piece of information you need to have not only a successful procedure but also a short and stress-free recovery period.

What to Ask (Yourself) before the Consultation

We hope that this book has helped to inform you about the safety of today's modern cosmetic procedures and has also given you the confidence to responsibly choose the ones you want. We also hope that you've used this book as a preconsultation tool, so that you still have plenty of time to search within yourself to see if surgical or even nonsurgical procedures are right for you.

Remember, your face is the first thing that most people notice when they see you; no doubt it's the first thing you look at every morning when you get up and one of the last things you look at every night before you go to bed. You have to be happy with your face if you're going to be happy with your life.

Something has made you pick up this book, and if you're still along for the ride, you've read 90 percent of it. This tells us that you're pretty sure about the desire for some type of cosmetic procedure, so logically, the next step is an initial consultation with the cosmetic specialist of your choice. We urge you not to let this critical opportunity pass by as nothing more than a routine visit to the doctor; it's not. You should consider this a fact-finding mission, a true opportunity to satisfy yourself that having a cosmetic procedure is the right thing for you and that you've found just the right doctor to perform it.

Following are the questions you should be asking yourself even before you go to the initial consultation.

Why Am I Really Having This Procedure Done?

Ask yourself this question—not just the generic reason you give everybody else, but the one deep down in your heart. Is it to reverse the signs of aging—or to look like your favorite celebrity? Any specialist can help you to turn back the hands of time and rediscover the vigor and fullness of your youthful skin; no doctor can perform a procedure to make you look like someone else.

Make sure your expectations are realistic when you go into the initial consultation, not just when you're having the procedure done. This is one of those times when knowing what to expect will give you better results in the long run, because by asking yourself this question now, you'll be even more prepared to ask it of your doctor during the consultation.

Is My Treatment Therapeutic?

Most cosmetic treatments are strictly cosmetic. However, there are several types of treatments that are wholly or largely for therapeutic purposes. These include treatments to correct serious deformities, medical conditions, and problems arising from illness or injury. These types of procedures are considered therapeutic and may be covered by your health insurance policy.

Some common therapeutic treatments include:

- Septoplasty (repair of a deviated septum)
- Upper blepharoplasty (eyelid lifts), when used to correct vision problems
- Skin cancer reconstruction
- Facial paralysis and Bell's palsy treatments
- Nasal and facial fracture or trauma reconstruction

Have I Thought It All the Way Through?

We have tried to cover a lot of ground in this book, from the mental to the physical to the social to the financial costs of having surgical and nonsurgical cosmetic procedures done on your face. We want you to be prepared before your procedure, to think it all the way through before actually going through with it.

Talk to your friends, your family, and your coworkers; ask around and get the opinions of those whom you love and trust the most. We want you to be comfortable with your decision, and the best way to do that is with some serious soul-searching before you ever meet your doctor.

The most important person, however, is you. You have to feel comfortable with your decision. Don't feel pressured by others—or by your doctor—to have something done. Conversely, if you feel strongly about a certain procedure when others don't, remember that it's *your* face. Read this book and discuss your concerns with your physician; if your concerns are within reason, then by all means go ahead with what you want.

Do I Have Enough Time to Devote to a Proper Recovery?

Every procedure has some recovery time involved, no matter how major or minor it might seem on the surface. Even if it is only a three- or four-day recovery time, your job, your family, or social pressures might not give you enough time to recover properly.

Consult your personal schedule and know in advance when is the best time for you to have your procedure. Be honest with yourself; don't be pressured into doing something just because it's summer or you have a long weekend coming up. Be patient and persistent in scheduling the right procedure at the right time. Your doctor can help you to schedule the procedure weeks to months in advance.

Do I Really Feel Healthy Enough to Go Through with This?

There is a time and a place for all things; cosmetic procedures are no different. If you are not in the best condition, if you have just had surgery or experienced an illness, or if you are just not feeling your best, it isn't the right time for you to have the procedure.

If you are having a major procedure performed, make sure that your physician asks you to obtain appropriate lab work, chest X-ray, electrocardiogram, and a medical clearance by your primary care physician or cardiologist. This is extremely important in order to avoid any major adverse event. If your physician tells you that a mini-face-lift or some other "minor" procedure is "no big deal," think twice about having him or her perform that procedure on you.

Will I Feel Complete without This Surgery?

We've all seen pictures of celebrities who seem to have some kind of addiction to the surgeon's scalpel, and we can't help but wonder sometimes if there might be something just a little addictive about changing our looks with cosmetic procedures.

Although we won't deny that there are people who seem to have one procedure after another, most of us don't notice the vast majority of people who appropriately have one or two procedures, quit there, and are perfectly happy with the results. We don't believe that plastic surgery is addictive, and we wouldn't work on someone who we thought had a problem of having too many procedures. There are, however, some individuals who have an obsessive-compulsive disorder or body dysmorphic syndrome (see sidebar) who are never happy with their looks or the outcome of cosmetic procedures.

Will There Be a Consultation Fee?

Most high-quality physicians will have a consultation fee to discuss potential cosmetic procedures. It is very important, however, that you don't get caught up in whether a physician has a consultation fee. It is your face that we are talking about, so don't count out doctors who charge a consultation fee. On the

BODY DYSMORPHIC DISORDER

Do you see yourself as others do? For that matter, do you see yourself as the tape measure, the scale, or your clothes sizes "see" you? Recently, a woman with severe anorexia nervosa went on *Dr. Phil* to discuss her eating disorder. Before the taping, she broke down and worried that Dr. Phil would think she was fat. At the time, she weighed just over sixty pounds, so to everyone in the audience, she was obviously far, far too thin—nearly skeletal. Yet her body image was such that she still felt fat.

This is an extreme case of a skewed body perspective, of course, but many people suffer from a less severe form called body dysmorphic disorder, or BDD. BDD manifests itself in people who have a severe disparity between how they think they appear and how they really look. For instance, someone might think that his head is far too big or too small for his frame, and another might think that she is much fatter than the scale or even her dress size indicates. These beliefs persist despite the physical measurements taken by a doctor.

In such cases, BDD can make these individuals seek plastic surgery to "correct" what they perceive to be wrong with their bodies. We have all seen pictures of people who have had dozens of surgeries to alter their bodies, but since their BDD is so severe, it becomes like a tiger chasing its tail: no matter how many surgeries are performed, one more is always necessary to look "just right." If you think you have either mild or severe BDD, consult a psychologist or a psychiatrist before consulting a plastic surgeon.

other hand, many amazing physicians also have complimentary consultations. Be wise, and if you think that you have found the right physician, go to see him or her regardless of a fee. Do diligent research, and if you are happy with everything else about that doctor's practice, don't let the consultation fee prohibit you from using a perfectly good physician.

Once you choose a doctor for your procedure, most will

require a deposit when you schedule a date for the procedure. Typically, this amount is then applied to the cost of your surgery.

What to Ask before the Procedure

All aspects of your procedure are different and, as such, require a different set of questions. The questions you ask before the initial consultation are vital and important, but they are not the same questions that you should ask after the consultation. Here are specific questions to ask after the consultation and before the cosmetic procedure itself.

How Much Will It Cost?

You will want to know before you have the procedure what fees you will be responsible for, and this is generally discussed during the initial consultation. However, as the time draws near for the procedure, it is never a bad idea to ask again.

This is especially useful if you are making payment arrangements with the physician's office and/or if you require various forms and releases signed by the medical office. At the very least, you want to know what you are responsible for and when, so that both your budget and your relationship with your trusted medical physician remain intact.

How Much Will My Insurance Cover?

Since most cosmetic procedures are elective and are not considered necessary by the average insurance company, it is important to know beforehand that you might not be reimbursed for the procedure. If the surgery is for medical reasons, your doctor can provide the proper forms to the insurance company, but it is important to deal with this beforehand so that you are not expecting something to be reimbursed when in all likelihood it might not be.

Where Will the Surgery Take Place?

Many of our procedures are done either in the office or as an out-patient procedure at an ambulatory surgical center or a local hospital. No doubt your experience will be the same. However, you will want to know exactly where the procedure will take place, how long it will take, and when you will be released, because most people need someone to drive them home and often to care for them during the first twenty-four to seventy-two hours after the procedure.

How Long Will the Procedure Take and What Are the Risks?

Most procedures we are involved in take less than a few hours to complete, but depending on the severity and the possible combination of your procedures, it could take more or less time. Your physician will be able to tell you exactly how much time your procedure will take (or at least give you a range) and, just as important, what to expect after the procedure is finished.

Every surgery has risks; knowing them ahead of time and taking the proper precautions is the best way to avoid them. Discuss frankly with your doctor what risks are involved and what to expect before, during, and after the surgery.

How Long Will It Take to Recover?

Many of our procedures take less than a week to recover from, and neither of us is a big fan of any procedure from which it takes longer than two weeks to recover. When discussing recovery times with your doctor, be open and honest about your threshold for pain as well as a realistic estimate of how much time off you can take. Don't be discouraged if you have to wait a few months or weeks to have the procedure done so that you can have more time for recovery, if necessary.

What Kind of Anesthesia Will My Doctor Use?

Based on the severity and length of the procedure itself, your doctor will consult a trained anesthesiologist to determine the right anesthesia for you. Your surgery will be performed using one of the following types of anesthesia:

- **Local anesthesia.** Here only a small portion of the patient's body, such as the eyelids or the lips, is numbed to prevent pain.
- **Regional anesthesia.** Here anesthesia is injected near a bundle of nerves to prevent pain, similar to the epidural that women are given before childbirth and the numbing shots that you receive in the dentist's office.
- **Intravenous sedation.** This is "twilight" anesthesia—another name for it is *conscious sedation*. The patient is neither fully conscious nor fully unconscious but is instead somewhere in between.
- **General anesthesia.** Here the patient is put and kept under anesthesia during the entirety of the procedure.

What Should I Do to Prepare for Plastic Surgery?

Your doctor will provide you with a checklist of things you should do before surgery If he or she doesn't, ask for one, or bring a notebook or ask for a sheet of paper and make a list for yourself. A good list will include all of the things you shouldn't do before the procedure—and how long beforehand you should stop—such as smoking, eating, drinking, or taking aspirin. It will tell you when you may resume the prohibited activities, and it will also include the things you *should* do beforehand, such as get a good night's rest and be at the doctor's office an hour early.

About two weeks before your procedure, we recommend that you get a list of medications that your physician does not want you to take. Every doctor has a different philosophy, but most physicians will want you to do the following:

- Stop taking aspirin and products that contain nonsteroidal anti-inflammatory drugs (NSAIDs), such as ibuprofen (Advil, Motrin) and naproxyn (Aleve, Naprosyn).
- If you are on blood thinners such as Coumadin, you should work with your physician to stop the medication in a controlled manner.
- Stop taking *all* vitamins (especially vitamins A, C, and E) and herbal supplements (such as St. John's wort);
- Stop smoking, and avoid all products that contain nicotine (such as patches, inhalers, and snuff or dip).
- Obtain appropriate lab work, an electrocardiogram, a chest X-ray, and a physical examination by your primary care physician.

In addition to being generally unhealthy and increasing the risk of aging in the face, smoking has been proven to inhibit both the amount of oxygen received by the skin and the flow of blood through the body. Both blood and oxygen are vital to the recovery process. Smoking has the potential to interfere with the face's healing process and to increase the risk of infection and skin necrosis (dead skin).

What to Ask before You Are Released

A lot happens after the procedure is finished but before you are released. There are bandages and ointments and lotions to consider, nurses to consult, and effects of anesthesia to overcome.

To delve more deeply into this topic, and considering the fact that you might be woozy after your procedure, we want to give you two caveats:

1. You should also ask these questions before your procedure.
2. Have a friend bring along these questions to ask in your stead after the procedure.

Following are the questions you should be most concerned about after your procedure is finished.

Will I Go Home after Surgery, and Can I Go Alone?

Most cosmetic procedures are done on an outpatient basis, which means that you will come into the surgical center and leave the same day. Typically, you will be monitored after your procedure and while you're coming out of the anesthesia; then, once it is determined that you are awake and aware, you will be released from the surgical center or hospital with instructions to return the next day to monitor your progress.

This means that although you will be able to get to the surgery yourself, you will need someone to drive you home, stay with you overnight, and drive you back the next day for your appointment. In total, you will need someone to be with you for forty-eight to ninety-six hours after surgery. We recommend that you have the same person drive you home from the procedure and back the next day; this person can also be your liaison with the doctor's office should anything go wrong.

Most cosmetic procedures are done on an outpatient basis, which means that you will come into the surgical center and go out the same day.

Occasionally, individuals from out of town may elect to stay in nearby aftercare facilities in order to be that much closer for the next day's postoperative visit. In this case, a nurse is present in the facility and will take care of all of the basic postoperative matters.

How Soon Will I Be Able to Resume Normal Physical Activity?

Depending on the procedure, you will be back to normal physical activity in three to five days. For some, this may include light household chores, driving, shopping, and socializing. Others may be able to go to work after a week. Check with your doctor first, but in general, all of this should be fine.

For any sort of exercise, however, we recommend waiting at least three weeks. The increase in blood pressure that is a result of strenuous physical exercise could affect the recovery time from your procedure, so it is best to play it safe.

Many of our patients are eager to know how soon they can wear makeup again. Generally speaking, you can start wearing makeup about one week after your procedure.

12

The Future Is Beautiful

The features of
our face are
hardly more than
gestures which
have become
permanent.

—MARCEL PROUST

What will the future hold for facial rejuvenation? Robotic surgeons? Lotions instead of needles? Lasers instead of knives? A better question might be this: What *won't* the future hold? As modern technology catches up with demand, attaining a more youthful and attractive appearance will not only get easier, it will be cheaper and accessible to millions of people all around the world.

We have been fortunate enough to watch the fields of dermatology and facial plastic surgery grow by leaps and bounds during our careers; we can only imagine what might develop in the next few decades as new products and procedures continue to astound and impress us with their ingenuity and efficacy. What's most amazing is the availability of rejuvenation for all ages and income brackets. Also impressive is the amount of information that is available today, so that readers like you can make wise, informed, and educated decisions about the future of your own face. No longer is the doctor an all-wise, all-seeing being who tells instead of listens. The encouraging new trend of doctors and patients as partners is encouraging on both sides of the desk, for you as well as your doctor.

As you can see, the future of facial rejuvenation fascinates us as much as, or perhaps even more than, the present. In this chapter we will try to present some educated predictions as we peer into the cosmetic crystal ball.

Changes in Aesthetic Ideals

Presently, most facial rejuvenation is done on a somewhat "per defect" basis. A patient sees a problem and goes to the doctor to get it fixed, with little or no counseling on what fixing that particular issue—a nose, perhaps, or a sagging brow—will mean to the appearance of the rest of the face.

We think that the future will usher in a more unified approach, with one of two possible goals: return of the face to age thirty or so, or revising the face to a more realistic ideal to which the patient can aspire. Suggestions for the ideal might arise from such sources as the Marquardt mask (see chapter 1). Does this sound like science fiction? We think it is gradually coming.

Will It Be Needle or Knife?

Once upon a time there was only one type of face-lift. Today, as we have written, there is a variety of modern face-lifts, and most of them come with the recommendation of fillers as complementary procedures. Is the face-lift going the way of the dinosaurs?

This is not entirely likely, but the future will undoubtedly bring an increasing emphasis on facial volume restoration and contouring with fillers (including fat) and less of an emphasis on surgery; however, the latter will still be the best, and sometimes the only, solution for loose neck skin (laxity). Volume restoration will evolve from art to science with clear results.

We believe that volume restoration will become more of an ideal as people recognize that firm and full, not strained or tight, is the new aesthetic. This can only be a good thing, because we will see less noticeable or surprised-look face-lifts and more natural procedures in which both doctor and patient are happy with the results. We envision the use of fillers to produce vectors that will adjust the skin to compensate for laxity lines that have resulted from the aging process.

Skin Care's New Levels of Efficacy

We expect home skin-care systems to include devices that increase the penetration of bioactive ingredients, making them less dependent on vehicles. Office procedures will do the same, but at much greater penetration levels. One recent example is an unpublished study on the Fraxel laser, which shows a sevenfold increase in the absorption of topical vitamin C that is applied after the laser procedure.

What will this mean for you? Ideally, you will make fewer trips to the doctor's office and will take more responsibility for and control of your own skin-care regimen. What excites us about this foreseeable trend is that by the time people do come to our offices, they will already be well versed in caring for their skin—both preop and postop.

Cosmeceuticals will broaden their antioxidant capacity by simultaneously dealing with several oxidative pathways. A particular dosage of skin-care products (such as application three times per week) may be recommended in some cases. Deeper penetration of skin-care products in combination with new powerful berry-derived antioxidants provide a major step forward.

Robotic Surgery

Will there ever come a time when *Star Trek*–like metal, rubber, and plastic hands work on your face? We don't know, but the precedent certainly exists. Robotic surgery has already revolutionized prostate and abdominal surgery.

We foresee a future in which facial surgery can be performed, at least in part, by programmed devices that eliminate surgical skill variations and operation fatigue. This will mean better results for you, because differences in doctor skill are reduced, and so are the ill effects of fatigue on such intricate operations.

Longer-Lasting Effects

In the future—and perhaps even in the near future—the relatively short duration of the Botox effect will undoubtedly be challenged by longer-lasting muscle paralyzers. These "next generation" toxins will increase the duration of wrinkle-free skin while decreasing the number of times you'll have to undergo the procedure.

Antidotes to Fillers

Presently, hyaluronidase can be used to reverse the effects of hyaluronic acid fillers such as Restylane and Juvéderm. This trend has allowed physicians to utilize the products with more confidence, because adverse events can be reversed. Steroids have also been injected into allergic lumps to reduce the side effects. We believe that in the future, more antidotes will be developed as the market continues to gain momentum.

Will Age Be Just a Number?

We foresee a future in which age—that is, your chronological age—will no longer be the only criterion for youth. Instead, your biological age will be viewed as more important in the long run, and the cocktail-party question may be "What is your chromosomal profile?" rather than "How old are you?" Different people clearly age at different biological rates depending on genetics and environmental influences.

We must learn to see ourselves in relation to our futures and not just as bodies in a vacuum. In other words, as people make wiser eating choices, as the dangers of smoking and drinking become more pronounced, and as doctors, diet, exercise, and prescription drugs do a better job of keeping us alive longer, we must learn to look how we feel.

We believe that the practice of facial rejuvenation will become increasingly important in future generations as older Americans yearn to look younger—but not at any cost. By demanding and using better, longer-lasting, and more trusted products and procedures, we can all look and feel younger.

FDA Studies

The government might decide to do the obvious: have the FDA do all drug and device approval studies using a sitting body of experts with funding by the company applying for approval. The process will then be more efficiently performed, of shorter duration, and perhaps less expensive to corporate America.

Presently FDA studies are done outside of the FDA under essentially the supervision of the company applying for approval; the data are later provided to the FDA. This potentially corrupts the integrity of the process and, at the least, reduces its efficiency.

Next-Generation Tightening Devices

In the next decade, we are likely to see tightening devices that will work on par with limited facial surgery. The technology is rapidly evolving, and billions of dollars are being spent in research labs to move the science forward. In fact, we can very realistically imagine a day when injectable volume restoration, skin lasers, and tightening devices will be the cornerstone of facial rejuvenation.

Customized Facial Implants

Implantech, one of the pioneers of facial implants, has developed custom-made facial implants from CT scans to correct facial defects due to trauma or congenital deformities. New developments in symmetry will usher in an era of change that many of our patients will welcome like nothing else.

Dr. William Binder has utilized this facial implant technology and has applied it for individuals who desire facial rejuvenation. We envision that this type of technology will become a more powerful and utilized technique in the field of aesthetic surgery to address significant facial atrophy, such as gauntness, hollow cheeks, and even "papery" skin. As the technology advances, it is likely to take the guesswork out and make the effects of atrophy a thing of the past for many people.

The ramifications will make custom implants a new and viable option for those who are seeking facial rejuvenation to increase fullness, determine shape, and even define features in a way that will be more natural-looking or, at the very least, more personal to the patient than they are today.

An issue at hand is the need to understand the end points that we are trying to achieve in correcting the aging process.

Stem Cells: The Magic Cure-All?

Much has been said of stem cell research in recent years, but what does it really mean? What are stem cells, where are they found, and how can they be used? Might stem cell research have applications for plastic surgery, dermatology, and the field of facial rejuvenation? The National Institutes of Health refer to stem cells this way:

> Stem cells have the remarkable potential to develop into many different cell types in the body. Serving as a sort of repair system for the body, they can theoretically divide

without limit to replenish other cells as long as the person or animal is still alive. When a stem cell divides, each new cell has the potential to either remain a stem cell or become another type of cell with a more specialized function, such as a muscle cell, a red blood cell, or a brain cell.

Think of stem cells as your body's way of remaking spare parts in your time of need. This is a slight oversimplification, but the very practical, timely hope for stem cell research is that instead of using synthetics in the future, we can use our own body's cells to regenerate muscles, skin, and even bone.

Although the practical application of stem cell research in plastic surgery and dermatology may still be a few years away, we'll go out on a limb and predict that you'll be seeing these procedures performed within a decade rather than the twenty to twenty-five years that most other researchers claim. The field of plastic surgery is playing a central role in this research.

In fact, plastic surgery has become a critical tool not only in the harvesting of stem cells but also in their testing and utilization. Adipose tissue-derived stem cells, or ADSCs, are basically stem cells that are derived from the fat taken out during liposuction procedures.

According to researchers at the Pennington Biomedical Research Center in Baton Rouge, Louisiana, "Adipose tissue has proven to serve as an abundant, accessible, and rich source of adult stem cells with multipotent properties suitable for tissue engineering and regenerative medical applications." Dr. Michael Miller, a member of the Plastic Surgery Educational Foundation (PSEF), explains as follows:

Stem cells obtained from fat during liposuction have the potential to develop into various kinds of body tissue such as bone, cartilage, muscle, and nerve cells. While similar stem cells can be obtained from bone marrow, liposuction may provide a larger quantity of stem cells [that are] more easily obtained. There is great potential for new therapies based on stem cell technology, however, significant obstacles exist.

Although ADSCs have revolutionized the way that stem cells are collected, that's only half the story. Collection is one thing, but implementation is another. People want to know which surgical and nonsurgical procedures can be enhanced, or eventually even replaced, by the benefits of stem cell research.

HealthDay reporter Steven Reinberg explains how many of us see the potential use of stem cells in our profession: "Using the person's own stem cells, plastic surgeons would create and shape implants from natural body tissue, instead of turning to the synthetic implants used in plastic surgery today." The caveat, of course, is that we're not cloning ourselves or regrowing parts we're not satisfied with or have lost, like a lizard growing back its tail. In the foreseeable future, the stem cells designed for an implant will still need a medium in which to grow.

In a study reported in *HealthDay*, researcher Jeremy J. Mao, director of the Tissue Engineering Laboratory at the University of Illinois at Chicago, placed stem cells into Hydrogel, "a U.S. Food and Drug Administration–approved substance that can be molded into any shape or size, mimicking the natural environment in which fat cells grow in the body. We found that the fatty tissue we created held its shape. This approach, down the road, will be useful for soft tissue reconstruction procedures."

A Japanese study used ADSCs to help women retain their natural breast shape after a lumpectomy. According to reporter Judy Peres in a December 15, 2007, story in the *Chicago Tribune*, "In the new study, doctors suctioned fat from each patient, usually from her abdomen or hips. They extracted stem cells from half the fat, then mixed the cells in with the remaining fat and injected it into the lumpectomy site. The hope is that the stem cells and other 'helper cells' will keep the transplanted tissue alive."

How did the trials work out? Says Peres: "The lead investigator, Dr. Keizo Sugimachi, reported at the San Antonio Breast Cancer Symposium that the procedure was safe and well-tolerated in all 21 subjects, with no signs of rejection. There was a significant improvement in breast volume, and eight months later most of the women were satisfied with the outcome."

Stem Cell Banking

Even though much of the research on stem cells is still in its early trial phase, many forward-thinking doctors are already seeing applications for the future. Since many view stem cells as the body's own source code for genetic reconstruction, it only makes sense that we would want to store as many such cells as we can for the future. Hence our industry's latest trend: stem cell banking.

Stem cell banking has great potential and implications for the future. Individuals can develop a personal stem cell "savings account" from their own liposuction procedures. Furthermore, as science advances and as technology catches up, and as more stem cells procedures become formal options (we predict these will start showing up in a decade or so), the patient will already have a stored source of his or her own stem cells with stem cell banking.

Your Physician's Role in the Future

Unfortunately, everything is not rosy in our crystal ball. There are likely to be two divergent trends in the future:

1. **Less specializing, more generalizing.** The core aesthetic specialties (plastic surgery, facial plastic surgery, dermatology, and oculoplastic surgery) will continue to deliver first-rate care as cross-training and educational tools grow by leaps and bounds. Not so long ago, most plastic surgeons hid their secrets from one another; today, most meetings flourish with multispecialty discussions about difficult subjects.
2. **The unqualified may heed the call.** The economic incentives of aesthetic medicine and declining medical reimbursements will continue to force physicians far removed from their core training to perform aesthetic procedures. This trend is not likely to be in the best interest of people, unless a more broad-based medical school and postgraduate training is incorporated into physician education.

Final Words about the Future

We hope that you've enjoyed our tour of the future of facial rejuvenation. The important thing to remember is how these changes will affect you. Just as we've tried to educate you throughout this book, it is important that you continue to educate yourself as the future becomes the present.

Stay informed. We don't necessarily recommend that you begin subscribing to the same medical journals and attending the same annual conferences that we do, but pay attention when you see or hear some breaking news story about a product or a procedure. Write down the name or follow the link to the Web site and do some additional research on your own. Find out the name of the procedure, its availability, and its cost and other such pertinent information, and ask your facial rejuvenation specialist about it. Does he or she recommend it or, for that matter, even know about it?

The future is bright, but don't wait for the trends to become so common that they're passé before you act on them. We see a shining future ahead for all of our patients, and we continue to urge them to act on their own, not only to care for their faces today but also to stay informed about the implications of the future and what it may mean for facial rejuvenation tomorrow.

Acknowledgments

The authors want to thank Nathalie Foo for her expert and untiring help in preparation of the manuscript. Our thanks to Rusty Fischer, whose considerable assistance with the preparation of this work was invaluable. Thanks go to our team at John Wiley & Sons, Christel Winkler and Lisa Burstiner, for believing in our work. Our deep appreciation to Tracie Souve for her editorial input. Finally, we thank the individual who made sure that our intentions became a reality, ushering our work from a proposal to a book on the shelves, Sharlene Martin, our cherished agent.

Index

Page numbers in *italics* refer to illustrations.